PocketRadiologist™
Cardiac
Top 100 Diagnoses

PocketRadiologist™
Cardiac
Top 100 Diagnoses

Thomas J Brady MD
Director, Cardiac Radiology, Massachusetts General Hospital
LL Robbins Professor of Radiology, Harvard Medical School
Boston, Massachusetts

Thomas M Grist MD
Professor of Radiology & Medical Physics
Vice Chair, Research & Education
Chief of Magnetic Resonance Imaging
University of Wisconsin-Madison
Madison, Wisconsin

Sjirk J Westra MD
Pediatric Radiologist, Massachusetts General Hospital
Associate Professor of Radiology, Harvard Medical School
Boston, Massachusetts

Stephan Wicky MD
Director, Clinic Cardiovascular Radiology
Vascular Radiology, Massachusetts General Hospital
Instructor of Radiology, Harvard Medical School
Boston, Massachusetts

Suhny Abbara MD
ISMRM / Nycomed Amersham Fellow in MRI
Division of Cardiac Radiology
Massachusetts General Hospital, Harvard Medical School
Boston, Massachusetts

With contribution by: *Paul Finn MD, Jeffrey J Hebert MD, Jude M Longo MD, Scott Pereles MD, Kris R Pillai MD, Theodore J Shinners MD, David Sosnovik MD*

With 200 drawings and radiographic images

Drawings: *Lane R Bennion MS, Richard Coombs MS James A Cooper MD, Jill Rhead MA*
Image Editing: *Ming Q Huang MD, Danielle Morris, Melissa Petersen*

Medical Text Editing: Richard H Wiggins III MD

AMIRSYS™

W. B. SAUNDERS COMPANY
An Elsevier Science Company

AMIRSYS™

A medical reference publishing company

First Edition

Text - Copyright Thomas J Brady MD 2003

Drawings - Copyright Amirsys Inc 2003

Compilation - Copyright Amirsys Inc 2003

First Printing: November 2002

Composition by Amirsys Inc, Salt Lake City, Utah

Printed by K/P Corporation, Salt Lake City, Utah

ISBN: 0-7216-0678-4

Preface

The **PocketRadiologist**™ series is an innovative, quick reference designed to deliver succinct, up-to-date information to practicing professionals "at the point of service." As close as your pocket, each title in the series is written by world-renowned authors. These experts have designated the "top 100" diagnoses or interventional procedures in every major body area, bulleted the most essential facts, and offered high-resolution imaging to illustrate each topic. Selected references are included for further review. Full color anatomic-pathologic computer graphics model many of the actual diseases.

Each **PocketRadiologist**™ title follows an identical format. The same information is in the same place - every time - and takes you quickly from key facts to imaging findings, differential diagnosis, pathology, pathophysiology, and relevant clinical information. The interventional modules give you the essentials and "how-tos" of important procedures, including pre- and post-procedure checklists, common problems and complications.

PocketRadiologist™ titles are available in both print and hand-held PDA formats. Currently available modules feature Brain, Head and Neck, Orthopedic (Musculoskeletal) Imaging, Pediatrics, Spine, Chest, Cardiac, Vascular, Abdominal Imaging and Interventional Radiology. 2003 topics will include Obstetrics, Gynecologic Imaging, Breast, and much, much more. Enjoy!

Anne G Osborn MD
Editor-in-Chief, Amirsys Inc

H Ric Harnsberger MD
Chairman and CEO, Amirsys Inc

Notice and Disclaimer

PocketRadiologist™
Cardiac
Top 100 Diagnoses

The diagnoses in this book are divided into 9 sections in the following order:

Congenital
Valvular
Pericardial
Neoplastic
Cardiomyopathy
Coronary Artery
Heart Failure
Hypertension
Vascular Disease

Table of Contents

Pericardial

Neoplastic

Cardiomyopathy

Table of Contents

Heart Failure

Hypertension

Vascular Disease

Table of Contents

PocketRadiologist™
Cardiac
Top 100 Diagnoses

CONGENITAL

Coarctation of Aorta

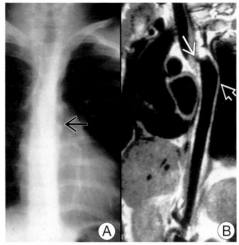

Coarctation of aorta. (A) Chest radiograph shows abnormal convex outline of aorta below aortic knob (arrow), the "3" sign. (B) Cardiac-gated sagittal-oblique T1 MR displays focal coarctation (arrow) distally to the left subclavian artery, with post-stenotic dilatation of proximal descending aorta (open arrow); compare with (A).

Key Facts
- Definition: Narrowing of the aortic lumen with obstruction to blood flow
- Classic plain film appearance: Rib notching, "figure 3" sign
- Category: Acyanotic, normal heart size and normal pulmonary vascularity
- Hemodynamics: Left ventricular (LV) pressure overload
- Major types
  - Preductal (infantile), juxtaductal and postductal (adult)
  - Simple (isolated) and complex (associated with other malformations)

Imaging Findings
General Features
- Best imaging clue: Focal aortic narrowing, presence of collaterals
Chest Radiography Findings
- Rib notching (above age 5 years)
- Post-stenotic dilatation of proximal descending aorta, "figure 3" sign
- LV hypertrophy: Rounded apex
- Esophagram: Impression by dilated descending aorta, "reversed 3" sign
Echocardiography Findings
- Imaging of aortic arch and branches in suprasternal long axis view
- Relationship of coarctation with patent ductus arteriosus (PDA)
- Doppler used to estimate gradient across coarctation
CT Findings
- CT angiography with 3D rendition depicts coarctation and collaterals
MR Findings
- Cardiac-gated T1WI (black blood)
  - Sagittal-oblique plane through aortic arch shows location of coarctation
  - Perpendicular views for cross-sectional diameter measurements
- Gradient-echo (GRE) cine (white blood)
  - In sagittal-oblique plane for anatomy
  - Length of systolic (dark) flow jet – hemodynamic significance

Coarctation of Aorta

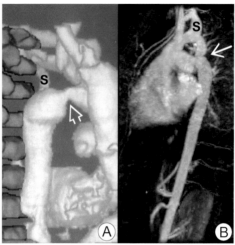

*Types of coarctation. (A) **Juxtaductal**, right lateral view from CT angiogram shows focal narrowing (arrow) in aortic arch proximally to subclavian artery (S). (B) **Postductal**, MR angiogram reveals shelf-like stenosis (arrow), poststenotic dilatation and large caliber of subclavian artery, due to significant collateral flow.*

- o Aortic regurgitation (bicuspid aortic valve)
- Phase-contrast MRA: For estimate of gradient and collateral flow
- 3D gadolinium MRA: For anatomy and depiction of collaterals

Cardiac Catheterization with Angiography Findings
- Direct measurement of gradient
- Balloon angioplasty

Imaging Recommendations
- Echocardiography for primary diagnosis in infancy
- Older child: MR for preoperative workup and postoperative surveillance for re-coarctation, aneurysms
- Catheterization reserved for gradient measurement and intervention

Differential Diagnosis

Hypoplastic Left Heart Syndrome
- Congestive heart failure in newborn
- Hypoplastic LV
- Ductus-dependent systemic perfusion
- Retrograde flow in hypoplastic ascending aorta

Interrupted Aortic Arch
- Flow to descending aorta via PDA

Pseudocoarctation
- Elongation with kinking of aorta without obstruction to blood flow

Takayasu's Arteritis
- Acquired inflammatory condition
- Acute phase: Aortic wall enhancement
- Chronic phase: Narrowing/occlusion of aorta and branch vessels

Coarctation of Aorta

Pathology
General
- General path comments
  - Frequently associated with bicuspid aortic valve (50%)
  - Other associations: Ventricular septal defect (VSD, 33%), PDA (66%), transposition, subaortic and mitral stenosis ("parachute" deformity, Shone's syndrome), Taussig-Bing anomaly, endocardial fibroelastosis
- Genetics
  - Usually sporadic
  - Associated with Turner's syndrome (20-36% have coarctation)
- Embryology
  - Postnatal contraction of fibrous ductal tissue in aortic wall
  - Abnormal fetal hemodynamics (e.g., hypoplastic left heart associated with preductal coarctation)
- Pathophysiology
  - Increase in systemic vascular resistance (left ventricular afterload)
  - Hypertension due to renal hypoperfusion
  - Congestive heart failure (newborn, associated complex heart disease)
  - LV hypertrophy
  - Development of collaterals to bypass the stenosis (internal mammary, intercostal, superior epigastric arteries)
- Epidemiology
  - Incidence: 2-6 per 10,000 live births
  - More common in males (2:1), Caucasians

Gross Pathologic, Surgical Features
- Focal shelf or waist lesion
- Diffuse narrowing of a segment of aortic arch (isthmus)
- Post-stenotic dilatation of descending aorta

Clinical Issues
Presentation
- Frequently asymptomatic, incidentally found
- Infancy: Congestive heart failure (due to associated anomalies)
- Older child, adult: Hypertension, diminished femoral pulses, differential blood pressure between upper and lower extremities (arm-leg gradient)
- Bacterial endocarditis

Treatment
- Resection and end-to-end anastomosis or interposition graft
- Prosthetic patch, subclavian flap aortoplasty
- Balloon angioplasty

Prognosis
- Re-coarctation (< 3%, higher when operated in infancy)
- Postoperative aneurysms (24% after patch angioplasty)
- Long-term survival decreased (late hypertension, coronary artery disease)

Selected References
1. Bogaert J et al: Follow-up of patients with previous treatment for coarctation of the aorta: Comparison between contrast-enhanced MR angiography and fast spin-echo MR imaging. Eur Radiol 10:1847-54, 2000
2. Riquelme C et al: MR imaging of coarctation of the aorta and its postoperative complications in adults: Assessment with spin-echo and cine-MR imaging. Magn Reson Imaging 17:37-46, 1999
3. Muhler EG et al: Evaluation of aortic coarctation after surgical repair: Role of magnetic resonance imaging and Doppler ultrasound. Br Heart J 70:285-90, 1993

Double Aortic Arch

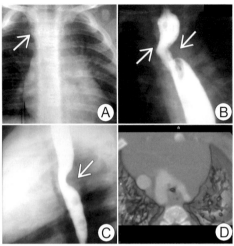

Double aortic arch in infant with stridor. Chest radiograph (A) and barium swallow (B,C) show mid-tracheal narrowing and characteristic lateral (B) and posterior (C) esophageal indentations (arrows) caused by both arches. The right arch (arrow, A) is the largest and more superior than the left. (D) CT image depicts both arches.

Key Facts
- Definition: Congenital arch anomaly characterized by persistence of both the left and right fourth aortic arches
- Classic plain film appearance: Trachea is deviated away from dominant arch and is narrowed in mid portion by indentations on either side
- Hemodynamics: No hemodynamic sequelae
- Most common symptomatic vascular ring
- Airway compression usually severe
- Presentation typically early in life

Imaging Findings
General Features
- Best imaging clue: Severe compression of trachea with evidence of right and left aortic arches
- On cross-sectional imaging, both left and right arches are identified arising from ascending aorta
- Each arch gives rise to a carotid and a subclavian artery
- Right arch more commonly larger and more superior/posterior than left
- Right arch typically runs behind esophagus to join left arch, to form left-sided descending aorta
- Part of left arch may be atretic but patent portions remain connected by fibrous band, forming a complete ring around trachea and esophagus
Chest Radiography Findings
- Prominent soft tissue on either side of the trachea
- Bilateral indentations on trachea, narrowing it in mid portion
- Right arch indentation commonly somewhat higher and more prominent than left
Barium Swallow Findings
- AP view: Bilateral indentations on upper esophagus at different levels
- Lateral view: Prominent horizontal posterior indentation

Double Aortic Arch

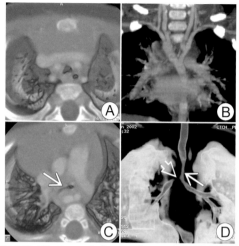

Double aortic arch. CT, same patient as previous page D. (A) Axial image shows symmetric takeoff of 4 arch vessels. (B) 3D image shows both arches joining posteriorly. Axial image (C) and airway rendition (D) show mid-tracheal narrowing by both arches (D, arrow) and right mainstem bronchomalacia (open arrow).

Echocardiography Findings
- Suprasternal notch view most helpful
- Two separate aortic arches, each giving rise to separate carotid and subclavian arteries (no right common brachiocephalic trunk)
- Often insufficient for preop diagnosis (does not show airway compression)

CT, MR Findings
- Axial and coronal images most helpful
- Four artery sign: Symmetric take-off of four aortic branches on axial image at thoracic inlet: 2 ventral carotids and 2 dorsal subclavians
- Two arches are seen, completely encircling trachea and esophagus, leading to severe mid-tracheal compression
- Smallest of two arches may be partially atretic
- 3D images are very helpful to demonstrate arch anatomy in relation to trachea

Imaging Recommendations
- Radiography followed by barium swallow
- Cross-sectional imaging (CT or MR) performed to confirm diagnosis and define anatomic variations for pre-surgical planning

Differential Diagnosis: Persistent Wheezing in Infant

Right Arch with Aberrant Left Subclavian Artery, Other Arch Abnormalities
- Generally not possible to differentiate without cross sectional imaging

Left Pulmonary Artery Sling
- Compression on posterior aspect of trachea and anterior aspect of esophagus on radiography

Innominate Artery Compression Syndrome
- Compression on anterior aspect of trachea, no esophageal compression

Nonvascular Masses
- Small middle mediastinal masses or larger anterior or posterior masses

Double Aortic Arch

Pathology

General

- General path comments
  - Airway narrowing due to extrinsic compression
  - Intrinsic abnormalities of tracheobronchial tree are frequently associated (tracheomalacia, complete cartilaginous ring)
- Genetics: No specific genetic defect identified
- Embryology
  - Persistence of the embryological right and left 4th aortic arches
- Pathophysiology
  - Severe airway and esophageal compression by vascular ring
- Epidemiology
  - Most common vascular ring anomaly (55%)

Gross Pathologic, Surgical Features

- True complete vascular ring with trachea and esophagus encircled
- Dominant right arch, left descending aorta: 75%
- Dominant left arch, right descending aorta: 25%
- Smallest of two arches may be partially atretic

Clinical Issues

Presentation

- Patients typically present early in life, often soon after birth
- Severe stridor, worsening with feeding
- Most common symptomatic vascular ring
- Typically not associated with other congenital abnormalities (isolated lesion)

Treatment & Prognosis

- Thoracotomy with division of the smaller of the two arches
- Determination of which arch is smaller on cross-sectional imaging will determine on which side thoracotomy is performed
- Up to 30% of patients may have persistent airway symptoms following initial surgical relief related to tracheomalacia, persistent extrinsic airway compression, or some combination of the two
- Some of these patients may benefit from a second operation, such as aortopexy, other vascular suspension procedures, or cartilaginous tracheal ring resection followed by reconstruction
- 11% of patients required a second operation to relieve airway symptoms

Selected References
1. Fleck RJ et al: Imaging findings in pediatric patients with persistent airway symptoms after surgery for double aortic arch. AJR 178:1275-9, 2002
2. Donnelly LF et al: The spectrum of extrinsic lower airway compression in children: MR imaging. AJR 168:59-62, 1997
3. Katz M et al: Spiral CT and 3D image reconstruction of vascular rings and associated tracheobronchial anomalies. J Comput Assist Tomogr 19:564-8, 1995

Right Aortic Arch

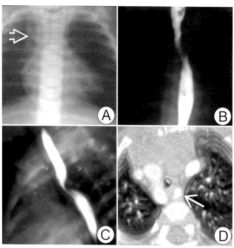

Right aortic arch. (A) Chest radiograph in infant with stridor: Right tracheal narrowing by arch (arrow). Barium swallow: Typical oblique (B) and posterior (C) indentations of aberrant left subclavian artery (LSA). Constricting left ductus ligament is likely. (D) CT in different infant: Right arch and aberrant LSA (arrow).

Key Facts
- Definition: Aortic arch courses over right main stem bronchus
- Classic plain film appearance: Aortic indentation on right of trachea, associated with prominent soft tissue density; trachea deviated to left
- Hemodynamics: Generally no hemodynamic disturbance
- Two major types
  - Mirror image branching pattern: Associated with cyanotic heart disease
  - Right arch with aberrant left subclavian artery (LSA): Isolated abnormality, not commonly associated with congenital heart disease
    - May be associated with airway compression: Left ligamentum arteriosum completes vascular ring, encircling trachea and esophagus

Imaging Findings
General Features
- Aortic arch located to right of trachea, coursing over right main stem bronchus

Chest Radiography Findings
- Aortic arch indentation on right of trachea
- Trachea is slightly deviated to the left
- More soft tissue density over right vertebral pedicle than over left
- Right-sided descending aorta line

Barium Swallow Findings
- Esophageal indentation only seen when aberrant LSA is present
- AP view: Oblique filling defect coursing from right-inferior to left-superior
- Lateral view: Posterior indentation
- Large posterior indentation: Aortic diverticulum of Kommerell

Echocardiography Findings
- Defines right arch, branching pattern (mirror image vs. aberrant LSA)

Right Aortic Arch

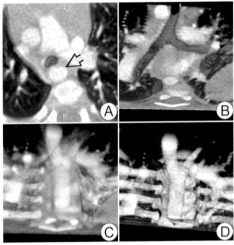

Right aortic arch, aberrant LSA, CT angiogram, same infant as previous page (D), who was asymptomatic. (A) Axial view shows takeoff of LSA from descending aorta (arrow). (B-D) Anterior views of cut-plane 3D renditions, various opacity settings, depict relationship of right arch and LSA with trachea, which is not stenosed.

CT, MR Findings
- Axial images define patency of arch segments, branching patterns
- Coronal images/reconstructions depict tracheal narrowing, if present

Imaging Recommendations
- Right arch with no airway compression: No further workup needed
- Right arch with airway compression: Look for aberrant LSA
  - Presence of constricting left ligamentum arteriosum can not be shown on imaging studies, but may be inferred → left thoracotomy needed

Differential Diagnosis

Double Aortic Arch with Dominant Right Arch
- Left arch often not well seen, atretic segment maintains fibrous continuity
- Characterized by tracheal narrowing, is always symptomatic (stridor)

Left Aortic Arch with Aberrant Right Subclavian Artery
- Mirror image of right aortic arch with aberrant LSA
- Oblique posterior esophageal indentation from left-inferior to right-superior
- Isolated abnormality, incidentally found (0.5% incidence in normal population), usually without airway compression
- Rarely symptomatic due to esophageal compression (dysphagia lusoria)

Pathology

General
- General path comments
  - All arch anomalies are a spectrum of the hypothetical double aortic arch model of Edwards
- Genetics
  - Right arch with mirror image branching: As with associated anomaly
  - Right arch with aberrant LSA: No specific genetic defect identified
- Embryology

Right Aortic Arch

- o Related to embryological persistence of the right 4th aortic arch
- o Retroesophageal (Kommerell) diverticulum: Remnant of embryonic left arch, connects to ductus ligament and gives rise to subclavian artery
- o Points of interruption of hypothetical double aortic arch (Edwards)
  - Normal development: Distal to right subclavian artery (RSA)
  - Right arch, mirror image branching: Distal to LSA
  - Right arch, aberrant LSA: Between left common carotid and LSA
  - Left arch, aberrant RSA: Between right common carotid and RSA
- Pathophysiology
  - o Airway compression only when complete tight vascular ring is present
  - o Symptomatic esophageal compression in the absence of airway compression is rare (dysphagia lusoria)
- Epidemiology
  - o Tetralogy of Fallot, pulmonary atresia/ventricular septal defect (VSD): 25% incidence right arch
  - o Truncus arteriosus: 30-40% incidence right arch
    - Cyanotic heart lesion with right arch: Tetralogy of Fallot is most likely, because tetralogy is far more common than truncus

Gross Pathologic, Surgical Features
- Constricting ligamentum arteriosum always opposite from dominant arch
- Posterior aortic diverticulum (Kommerell) at origin of aberrant subclavian artery may contribute to mediastinal crowding and airway compression

Clinical Issues
Presentation
- Right arch with aberrant LSA: Incidental finding, often asymptomatic
  - o May cause symptoms in infancy, provoked by airway infection (mucosal edema), improves with age and growth of child
  - o Posterior esophageal indentation by aberrant subclavian artery rarely causes dysphagia (lusoria)
  - o With constricting left ligamentum arteriosum: Congenital stridor
- Right arch with mirror image branching: Associated with cyanotic congestive heart disease (CHD)
Natural History
- Determined by natural history of cyanotic heart lesion, if associated
Treatment
- Right arch with aberrant LSA and constricting (symptomatic) left ligamentum arteriosum: Division of ligamentum via left thoracotomy
  - o Aortopexy may me needed additionally
  - o Associated complete cartilaginous tracheal ring: Resection and tracheal reconstruction and/or stenting may be needed additionally
- Otherwise dependent on associated congenital heart lesion
Prognosis
- Determined by prognosis of cyanotic heart lesion, if associated
- Tracheomalacia, residual stenosis and vascular compression are common after vascular ring repair, occasionally requiring additional surgery

Selected References
1. Donnelly LF et al: Aberrant subclavian arteries: Cross-sectional imaging findings in infants and children referred for evaluation of extrinsic airway compression. AJR 178:1269-74, 2002
2. Hopkins KL et al: Pediatric great vessel anomalies: Initial clinical experience with spiral CT angiography. Radiology 200:811-5, 1996
3. Lowe GM et al: Vascular rings: 10-year review of imaging. Radiographics 11:637-46, 1991

Pulmonary Sling

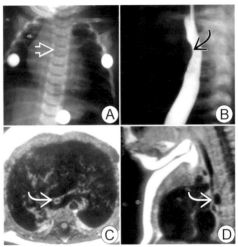

Pulmonary sling in infant with stridor. (A) Chest radiography shows distal tracheal compression (open arrow), left lung hyperinflation. (B) Barium swallow: Anterior indentation on esophagus (curved arrow). (C,D) Axial, sagittal T1WI shows left pulmonary artery sling surrounding & compressing distal trachea (curved arrows).

Key Facts
- Synonym: Aberrant left pulmonary artery
- Definition: Left pulmonary artery arises from the right, rather than the main pulmonary artery
- Classic plain film appearance: Asymmetric lung inflation, narrowing of distal trachea which is displaced towards the left
- Hemodynamics: Determined by associated cardiac anomaly
- It is the only vascular ring associated with asymmetric lung inflation
- Associated in 50% with other congenital lesions such as congenital heart disease
- Often associated with complete tracheal rings (50%)
- Typically presents early in life with severe stridor

Imaging Findings
General Features
- The left pulmonary artery forms a "sling" around the distal trachea as it passes leftward between the trachea and esophagus
- Only vascular ring to course between the trachea and esophagus (compresses trachea from behind and esophagus from front)

Chest Radiography Findings
- It is the only vascular ring associated with asymmetric lung inflation
- Lateral view: Round soft-tissue density between distal trachea and esophagus
- Posterior compression of the trachea, typically distally at the level of the distal trachea or carina
- Distal trachea or right main bronchus may be bowed anteriorly
- Low position of the left hilum

Pulmonary Sling

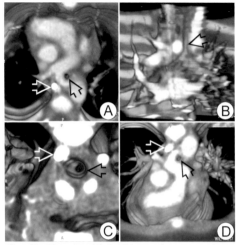

Pulmonary sling, 3D CT angio. (A) Axial image shows anomalous origin of left pulmonary art. Courses between esophagus (identified by nasogastric tube, white open arrow) & stenosed distal trachea (black open arrow). Cut-plane anterior (B), superior (C,D) views of 3D renditions depict distal tracheal narrowing by sling.

Barium Swallow Findings
- It is the only vascular ring that leads to an anterior indentation on the esophagus
- Trachea is compressed at same level from posteriorly

Echocardiography Findings
- Absence of normal pulmonary artery bifurcation
- Anomalous origin of left pulmonary artery from proximal right pulmonary artery
- Associated other cardiac anomalies

CT, MR Findings
- Cross-sectional imaging is needed to confirm diagnosis and delineate anatomy prior to surgery
- Pulmonary sling and tracheal compression typically best demonstrated on axial CT or MR images
- The left pulmonary artery arises from the right, rather than the main, pulmonary artery
- The left pulmonary artery forms a "sling" around the trachea as it passes leftward between the trachea and esophagus
- Degree of tracheal compression typically severe
- Distal trachea and carina often displaced to the left
- Often findings of coexisting congenital heart disease present
- When complete tracheal ring is present, the trachea will have a round (rather than oval) appearance with an abnormally small diameter

Differential Diagnosis

Middle Mediastinal Mass
- Lymphadenopathy
- Bronchogenic cyst

Pulmonary Sling

Midline Descending Aorta/Carina Compression Syndrome
- Descending aorta immediately anterior to spine, leading to "crowding" of mediastinum: Posterior compression on carina or left main stem bronchus
- May be isolated, or associated with right lung hypoplasia, arch anomalies

Pathology
General
- General path comments
  o Frequently associated with significant hypoplasia/dysplasia of distal trachea and main stem bronchi
- Genetics: No specific genetic defect identified
- Embryology
  o Agenesis or obliteration of the left sixth aortic arch, which normally forms the left branch pulmonary artery
  o Arterial supply of left lung via persistent primitive artery originating from right pulmonary artery
- Pathophysiology: Severe stridor secondary to
  o Compression of distal trachea, carina, main stem bronchi: Uneven inflation of the lungs (obstructive emphysema > atelectasis)
  o Associated tracheobronchomalacia
  o Associated intrinsic airway narrowing (complete cartilaginous rings)
Gross Pathological, Surgical Features
- The left pulmonary artery arises from the right, rather than the main, pulmonary artery
- The left pulmonary artery forms a "sling" around the trachea as it passes leftward between the trachea and esophagus
- It enters hilum of left lung posteriorly to left main stem bronchus
- Severe compression of distal trachea and right main stem bronchus
- Main stem bronchi have abnormally horizontal course ("inverted T"), with abnormal branching pattern to upper and lower lobes (more peripherally)

Clinical Issues
Presentation
- Presentation with stridor, "noisy breathing," apneic spells or recurrent pulmonary infections early in life
Treatment
- Surgical division of left pulmonary artery from its anomalous origin, with implantation to its normal location of origin, from main pulmonary artery
- Tracheobronchial reconstruction if there is a complete tracheal cartilaginous ring or other associated tracheobronchial malformation
Prognosis
- Less favorable than other vascular rings
  o High association with congenital heart disease
  o High incidence of intrinsic tracheobronchial anomalies, tracheomalacia

Selected References
1. Donnelly LF et al: The spectrum of extrinsic lower airway compression in children: MR imaging. AJR 168:59-62, 1997
2. Katz M et al: Spiral CT and 3D image reconstruction of vascular rings and associated tracheobronchial anomalies. J Comput Assist Tomogr 19:564-68, 1995
3. Dohlemann C et al: Pulmonary sling: Morphological findings, pre- and postoperative course. Eur J Pediatr 154:2-14, 1995

D-Transposition

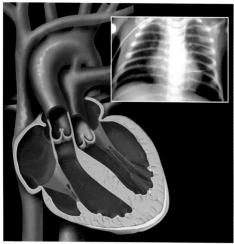

D-transposition of the great arteries. Drawing depicts anteriorly-placed aorta, connected via infundibulum to right ventricle, and posteriorly-placed pulmonary artery, directly connected to left ventricle. Flow admixture is possible via patent foramen ovale and ductus arteriosus. Insert: Typical chest radiograph in neonate.

Key Facts
- Synonym: Ventriculoarterial discordance with atrioventricular concordance
- Definition: Aorta arises from right ventricle (RV) and pulmonary artery (PA) arises from left ventricle (LV)
- Classic plain film appearance: "Egg-on-side" cardiomediastinal silhouette
- Category: Cyanotic, cardiomegaly, increased pulmonary vascularity
- Hemodynamics
  - RV connected with systemic circulation: Pressure overload
  - LV connected with pulmonary circulation: Volume overload
  - Incompatible with life without flow admixture: Patent foramen ovale (PFO), ventricular septal defect (VSD), patent ductus arteriosus (PDA)

Imaging Findings
General Features
- Best imaging clue: Great vessels lie parallel and almost in the same sagittal plane, with aortic valve in anterior position and slightly to the right (D-loop) of pulmonary valve
Chest Radiography Findings
- Cardiomegaly
- Narrow mediastinum ("egg-on-side")
- Increased pulmonary vascularity
Echocardiography Findings
- Segmental cardiac analysis: Identification of atria, ventricles, great arteries and their connections
- Identification of PFO, VSD, PDA
- Proximal coronary artery anatomy
CT Findings
- 3D CT angiography depicts abnormal ventriculoarterial relationship

D-Transposition

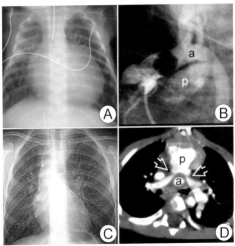

D-Transposition. (A) Chest radiograph: "Egg-shaped" heart, narrow mediastinum. (B) Angiogram: Reversed relationship between ascending aorta (a) and pulmonary artery (p). (C) Chest radiograph after Mustard repair: Abnormal great vessel orientation. (D) CT after arterial switch: Bilateral branch PA stenoses (arrows).

MR Findings
- Multiplanar cardiac-gated T1WI, GRE cine and 3D Gadolinium MRA
  - Segmental cardiac analysis of axial slices reveals atrioventricular concordance and ventriculoarterial discordance
  - Presence of PFO, VSD, PDA, pulmonary valve stenosis, subpulmonic stenosis
  - Useful to assess baffle obstruction after Mustard/Senning procedures

Cardiac Catheterization and Angiography Findings
- Only needed for Rashkind procedure (emergency balloon atrial septostomy)

Imaging Recommendations
- Echocardiography allows for complete preoperative diagnosis in majority
- CT or MRI for postoperative complications of PAs, atrial baffle

Differential Diagnosis

Complex Transposition
- Associated (sub-) pulmonary stenosis, VSD

Associated (Pre-ductal) Coarctation with PDA
- Small right ventricle, aorta; large left ventricle and PA

Pathology

General
- General path comments
  - Atria and ventricles are morphologically normal
  - Coronary anomalies are frequent
    - Right coronary artery dominance
    - Circumflex coronary artery originates from right coronary artery
    - Single coronary ostium
- Genetics

- o No genetic factors identified
- o Not associated with extracardiac malformations or chromosomal abnormalities
- Embryology
  - o Single embryological error: Faulty separation of aorta and pulmonary artery from primitive bulbus cordis (conotruncus)
  - o Heart is otherwise structurally normal
- Pathophysiology
  - o Complete separation of pulmonary and systemic circulations
  - o Survival dependent on admixture: PFO, VSD, PDA
- Epidemiology
  - o Incidence: 1 in 3000 live births
  - o 5% of congenital heart disease
  - o Males > females

Gross Pathologic, Surgical Features
- Infundibulum of RV connected to aortic valve, anterior and slightly to right of midline (D-loop)
- LV connected without infundibulum to pulmonary valve, posterior and slightly to left of aortic valve

Clinical Issues

Presentation
- Severe cyanosis not improving with oxygen, with little respiratory distress

Natural History
- Early death without communicating shunt
- Large VSD: Congestive heart failure in first weeks of life
- Patients with large VSD and (sub-) pulmonic stenosis have mild symptoms and may survive for years without treatment

Treatment
- Prostaglandin E_1 infusion to keep ductus arteriosus open
- Emergency balloon atrial septostomy (Rashkind procedure)
- Surgical early: Arterial switch with transposition of coronaries (Jatene)
  - o Late arterial switch not possible (pressure drops after birth in LV connected to pulmonary circulation, which is then no longer able to sustain systemic arterial pressures)
- Surgical late: Re-routing of venous flow in atria with pericardial baffle (Mustard) or reorientation of the atrial septum (Senning)

Prognosis
- Simple transposition: Good with early arterial switch
- Complication of arterial switch: Traction on branch PAs by anteriorly transposed main PA, leading to PA branch origin stenosis
- Long-term prognosis determined by potential coronary abnormalities
- Complex transposition: Dependent of associated anomalies
- Mustard/Senning procedures: RV failure, atrial thrombosis, arrhythmias

Selected References
1. Gutberlet M et al: Arterial switch procedure for D-transposition of the great arteries: Quantitative midterm evaluation of hemodynamic changes with cine MR imaging and phase-shift velocity mapping – initial experience. Radiology 214:467-75, 2000
2. Blakenberg F et al: MRI vs. echocardiography in the evaluation of the Jatene procedure. J Comput Assist Tomogr 18:749-54, 1994
3. Beek FJ et al: MRI of the pulmonary artery after arterial switch operation for transposition of the great arteries. Pediatr Radiol 23:335-40, 1993

L-Transposition

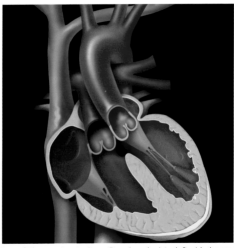

L-transposition of the great arteries. Drawing depicts left-sided ascending aorta, connected via infundibulum to left-sided trabeculated right ventricle, and right-sided pulmonary artery, directly connected to right-sided smooth-walled left ventricle. Note the commonly associated ventricular septal defect.

Key Facts
- Synonyms: Atrioventricular discordance and ventriculoarterial discordance, "congenitally corrected transposition" (misnomer)
- Definition: Inversion of ventricles and great arteries
- Classic plain film appearance: Straight upper left heart border
- Category: Dependent on associated anomalies
  - Ventricular septal defect (VSD, 60-70%): Acyanotic, increased pulmonary vascularity
  - Pulmonary outflow tract obstruction (30-50%): Cyanotic
  - Dysplasia, regurgitation and Ebstein's anomaly of left-sided atrioventricular (AV) valve: Pulmonary venous congestion/hypertension
  - Conduction abnormalities, heart block
  - Only 1% have no associated anomalies: True congenitally corrected transposition
- Hemodynamics
  - Right atrium connects via mitral valve to right-sided morphologically left ventricle (LV), which connects to pulmonary circulation
  - Left atrium connects via tricuspid valve to left-sided morphologically right ventricle (RV), which connects to systemic circulation
  - Hemodynamic sequelae dependent on associated anomalies

Imaging Findings
General Features
- Best imaging clue: Great vessels lie parallel and almost in the same coronal plane, with aortic valve in anterior position and slightly to the left (L-loop) of pulmonary valve
Chest Radiography Findings
- Straight left upper heart border

L-Transposition

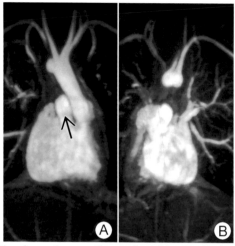

L-transposition. Consecutive coronal images of gadolinium MRA (A, B) in patient with complex cyanotic heart disease and double-outlet right ventricle demonstrate malposition of ascending aorta, located to the left of and parallel to the main pulmonary artery (arrow).

- Otherwise dependent on associated anomalies

Echocardiography Findings
- Segmental cardiac analysis: Identification of atria, ventricles, great arteries and their connections
- Continuity between right-sided mitral and pulmonary valve annulus
- Discontinuity between left-sided tricuspid and aortic valve annulus
- Abnormally straight, vertical course of interventricular septum

CT Findings
- 3D CT angiography depicts abnormal atrioventricular and ventriculoarterial relationships

MR Findings
- Multiplanar cardiac-gated T1WI and 3D gadolinium MRA for segmental cardiac analysis and anatomic evaluation
- Dobutamine stress GRE cine MRI for functional evaluation of RV

Cardiac Catheterization and Angiography Findings
- Defines ventricular inversion, abnormal atrioventricular and ventriculoarterial connections, VSD, pulmonary outflow tract obstruction, tricuspid valve dysfunction

Imaging Recommendations
- Echocardiography allows for complete preoperative diagnosis in majority
- CT or MRI as complementary test for more complex abnormalities

Differential Diagnosis

Congestive Heart Failure, Increased Pulmonary Blood Flow
- Isolated VSD, double inlet ventricle, tricuspid atresia with increased pulmonary blood flow, double outlet right ventricle with subaortic VSD

Cyanosis, Decreased Pulmonary Blood Flow
- Tetralogy of Fallot

L-Transposition

Pathology

General

- General path comments
  - Ventricular arrangement is not simply the mirror image of normal
  - Ventricles and great arteries form an L-loop (D-loop is normal)
  - Interventricular septum is more vertical than normal
  - Coronary distribution is mirror image of normal (right-sided coronary bifurcates into circumflex and anterior descending arteries)
- Genetics
  - No genetic factors or chromosomal abnormalities identified
  - Not commonly associated with extracardiac malformations
- Embryology
  - Primitive cardiac tube loops to the left (L-loop), leading to ventricular inversion and left-sided position of ascending aorta
- Pathophysiology
  - Determined by associated abnormalities: VSD, pulmonary stenosis, dysfunction of systemic AV valve
  - Late sequel: RV is not able to sustain systemic circulation
- Epidemiology
  - Incidence: 1 in 13,000 live births, 1% of congenital heart disease, males > females

Gross Pathologic, Surgical Features

- Right-sided morphologic LV connected without infundibulum to pulmonary valve, which is slightly posterior and to right of aortic valve
- Infundibulum of left-sided morphological RV connected to aortic valve, which is slightly anterior and to left of pulmonary valve (L-loop)
- Pulmonary artery and ascending aorta lie parallel in same coronal plane

Clinical Issues

Presentation

- Asymptomatic, incidental finding on chest radiograph
- Congestive heart failure (VSD, systemic AV valve dysfunction)
- Cyanosis (pulmonary outflow tract obstruction)
- Conduction disturbances: Bradycardia (heart block), tachydysrhythmia

Natural History

- Determined by presence of AV valve dysfunction

Treatment

- Surgical treatment focussed on associated abnormalities
  - VSD closure, LV to pulmonary artery conduit, tricuspid valvuloplasty
- Double switch operation to prevent late systemic ventricular (RV) failure

Prognosis

- Guarded due to progressive systemic AV valve and RV dysfunction after corrective surgery: 50% mortality after 15 years
- Patients with true congenitally corrected transposition may have a normal life expectancy

Selected References
1. Tulevski II et al: Usefulness of magnetic resonance imaging dobutamine stress in asymptomatic and minimally symptomatic patients with decreased cardiac reserve from congenital heart disease (complete and corrected transposition of the great arteries and subpulmonic obstruction). Am J Cardiol 89:1077-81, 2002
2. Reddy GP et al: Case 15: Congenitally corrected transposition of the great arteries. Radiology 213:102-6, 1999
3. Chen SJ et al: Three-dimensional reconstruction of abnormal ventriculoarterial relationship by electron beam CT. J Comput Assist Tomogr 22:560-8, 1998

Tetralogy of Fallot

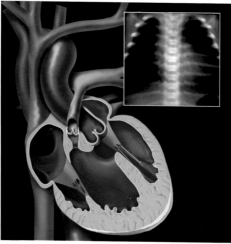

Tetralogy of Fallot. Drawing depicts subvalvular (infundibular) pulmonary stenosis, small pulmonary valve, large aortic valve overriding high ventricular septal defect right ventricular hypertrophy, and right-sided aortic arch. Insert: Chest radiograph in cyanotic infant: Boot-shaped heart, pulmonary oligemia, right arch.

Key Facts
- Definition: Infundibular right ventricular outflow tract (RVOT) stenosis, subaortic ventricular septal defect (VSD), overriding aorta and right ventricle (RV) hypertrophy
- Classic plain film appearance: "Boot-shaped" heart
- Category: Cyanotic, normal heart size, decreased pulmonary vascularity
- Hemodynamics
  - Outflow obstruction of right ventricle, leading to pressure overload
  - Balance between RVOT obstruction (classic Fallot; decreased pulmonary blood flow, cyanosis) and VSD ("pink" Fallot; normal or increased pulmonary blood flow, congestive heart failure)
  - Spectrum: "Pink" Fallot - classic Fallot - pulmonary atresia with VSD and multiple aorticopulmonary collateral arteries (MAPCAs)
- Tetralogy of Fallot is most common heart lesion with right aortic arch

Imaging Findings
General Features
- Best imaging clue: Infundibular stenosis of RVOT
Chest Radiography Findings
- Normal heart size
- Right-sided aortic arch in 25%
- RV hypertrophy, concave pulmonary artery segment: "Boot-shaped" heart = "coeur en sabot"
- Decreased pulmonary vascularity (pulmonary oligemia)
Echocardiography Findings
- Location VSD, additional muscular VSDs
- Degree of aortic override, position of arch
- Degree of RVOT obstruction, function of pulmonary valve
- Anatomy of branch pulmonary arteries (PAs)

Tetralogy of Fallot

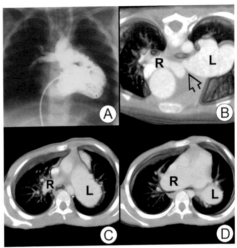

Variations of Fallot, (A) "Pink" Fallot, right ventricle injection: Simultaneous filling of aorta, normal caliber pulmonary arteries (PAs). (B) CT angiogram (CTA): Left PA origin stenosis (arrow), with poststenotic dilation. (C,D) CTA, absent pulmonary valve: Massively dilated PAs (R, L) compressing tracheobronchial tree.

CT Findings
- CT angiography with volume rendition depicts PA anatomy

MR Findings
- Cardiac-gated T1WI (axial views)
  - Preoperative definition of PA anatomy, PA stenosis
  - Postoperative PA anatomy, patency of Blalock-Taussig shunts
- Gradient-echo (GRE) cine in short axis
  - RV function, ejection fraction
- Phase-contrast MRA: For estimate of RV function, regurgitation fraction
- 3D gadolinium MRA: For anatomy and depiction PA anatomy and MAPCAs

Cardiac Catheterization and Angiography Findings
- Coronary anatomy
- PA branch stenosis: Balloon angioplasty with stent placement
- Anatomy/distribution of MAPCAs

Imaging Recommendations
- Initial diagnosis with echocardiography
- MRI or CTA for PA anatomy
- Cardiac catheterization for percutaneous interventions
- MRI in older child with poor acoustic window for functional assessment of postoperative pulmonary regurgitation and RV dysfunction

Differential Diagnosis

Pulmonary Atresia with VSD and MAPCAs

Tricuspid Atresia with VSD
- Muscular or membranous partition between right atrium and RV
- Obligatory shunting from right atrium → left atrium → LV → RV
- Decreased pulmonary flow → severe cyanosis at birth
- When associated with transposition increased pulmonary blood flow

Tetralogy of Fallot

Pathology

General
- Frequently associated
  o PA branch stenosis or hypoplasia
  o Absence of pulmonary valve: Severe pulmonary regurgitation → aneurysmal dilatation of PAs → tracheobronchial compression
  o Patent foramen ovale
  o Right-sided aortic arch with mirror image branching (25%)
  o Coronary anomalies: Left anterior descending (LAD) arising from right coronary and crossing RVOT, with implications for surgical repair
- Genetics
  o Associated with chromosomal abnormalities in 11% (chromosome 22)
  o Associated with other congenital anomalies in 16%; syndromal in 8%
- Embryology
  o Abnormal bulbotruncal rotation and septation
  o Primary hypoplasia of infundibular septum
- Epidemiology
  o Incidence: 3-5 per 10,000 live births
  o Fourth most common congenital heart anomaly
  o Most common cyanotic heart lesion

Clinical Issues

Presentation
- Varying degrees of cyanosis at birth
- Clubbing of fingers and toes
- Hypercyanotic spells, relieved by squatting
- Congestive heart failure (large VSD)
- After repair: Decreased exercise tolerance, RV dysfunction, arrhythmias
- Bacterial endocarditis, stroke due to paradoxical embolus to brain, hyperviscosity syndrome due to polycythemia

Natural History
- Ten percent of untreated patients live more than 20 years

Treatment
- Palliative shunt
  o Classic Blalock-Taussig shunt: End-to-side subclavian artery to PA (opposite from aortic arch)
  o Modified Blalock-Taussig shunt: Interposition of Gore-Tex graft
  o Central shunt: Ductus-like connection between aorta and PA
- Complete repair: Enlargement of RVOT, closure of VSD
  o With transannular patch: Postop pulmonary regurgitation

Prognosis
- Short term: Excellent results after early complete repair
- Long term: Determined by right ventricular diastolic dysfunction

Selected References
1. Holmqvist C et al: Pre-operative evaluation with MR in tetralogy of Fallot and pulmonary atresia with ventricular septal defect. Acta Radiol 42:63-9, 2001
2. Helbing WA et al: Clinical applications of cardiac magnetic resonance imaging after repair of tetralogy of Fallot. Pediatr Cardiol 21:70-9, 2000
3. Greenberg SB et al: Magnetic resonance imaging compared with echocardiography in the evaluation of pulmonary artery abnormalities in children with tetralogy of Fallot following palliative and corrective surgery. Pediatr Radiol 27:932-5, 1997

Truncus Arteriosus

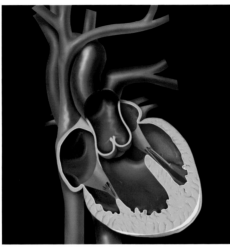

Truncus arteriosus. Drawing illustrates type 1 truncus with common truncal valve, overriding high ventricular septal defect, giving rise to aorta (note right aortic arch) and main pulmonary artery (which bifurcates into right and left branches). Cyanosis is due to flow admixture within the ventricles and the truncus.

Key Facts
- Synonym: Common arterial trunk
- Definition: Common arterial vessel arising from the heart, giving rise to aorta, pulmonary arteries (PAs) and coronary arteries
- Classic plain film appearance: Cardiomegaly, increased pulmonary vascularity, narrow mediastinum, right aortic arch
- Category: Cyanotic, cardiomegaly, increased pulmonary vascularity
- Hemodynamics
  - Both ventricles connected with pulmonary and systemic circulation
  - Flow admixture at ventricular septal defect (VSD) and within truncus
  - Postnatal drop in pulmonary vascular resistance → relative increase in pulmonary blood flow → volume overload of pulmonary circulation
- Truncus arteriosus is the heart lesion most commonly associated with right aortic arch (30-40%)
- Frequently associated with absent thymus (T-cell immunodeficiency) and absent parathyroid glands (neonatal tetany): DiGeorge syndrome

Imaging Findings
General Features
- Best imaging clue: Common arterial trunk arising from both ventricles
Chest Radiography Findings
- Cardiomegaly
- Active pulmonary vascular congestion
- Right aortic arch in 25%
- Narrow mediastinum due to thymic agenesis
Echocardiography Findings
- Common arterial trunk originating from both ventricles
- High (outlet) ventricular septal defect immediately below truncal valve
- Common truncal valve with 2, 3 or 4 cusps

Truncus Arteriosus

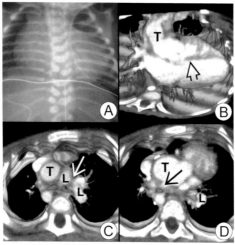

Type 3 truncus arteriosus. (A) Chest radiograph shows cardiomegaly and vertebral anomalies. Frontal (B) and axial (C, D) views of CT angiogram depict large truncus (T) overriding VSD (open arrow), right aortic arch, small right (black arrow) and larger left (L) pulmonary artery, which was surgically banded (white arrow).

Cardiac Catheterization with Angiography Findings
- Simultaneous opacification of aorta and pulmonary arteries

CT Findings
- CT angiography with 3D reconstruction shows relationship of branch pulmonary arteries with truncus

MR Findings
- Cardiac-gated T1WI in axial plane: Pulmonary artery anatomy
- Gadolinium-MRA: Global anatomy, patency of conduit

Imaging Recommendations
- Primary diagnosis made with echocardiography
- MRI/CTA for preoperative delineation of pulmonary artery anatomy
- MRI/CTA for postoperative assessment of conduit stenosis

Differential Diagnosis

Transposition of the Great Arteries
- Presents earlier in life with more severe cyanosis, ductus-dependent

Aorticopulmonary Window
- Congenital fenestration between separate ascending aorta and PA, with separate aortic and pulmonary valves

Pathology

General
- General path comments
  - Common outflow tract of both ventricles, over non-restrictive VSD
  - No separate outflow portion (infundibulum) of right ventricle
- Genetics
  - Strong association with deletion on the long arm of chromosome 22 (22q11 syndrome)
  - Associated with characteristic abnormal facies

Truncus Arteriosus

- o CATCH-22: Conofacial abnormality, absent thymus, hypocalcemia, heart defect
- Embryology
  - o Lack of separation of primitive bulbus cordis into aorta and pulmonary arteries
  - o Associated persistence of primitive aortic arches
- Pathophysiology
  - o Marked increase in pulmonary blood flow
  - o Cyanosis due to admixture
- Epidemiology
  - o Incidence: 2% of congenital cardiac anomalies

Gross Pathologic, Surgical Features
- Four main types
  - o Type 1: Separation of trunk into ascending aorta and main PA
  - o Type 2: Common take-off of branch PAs from trunk, with no main PA
  - o Type 3: Both branch PAs originate separately from posterolateral aspect of ascending aorta
  - o Type 4: "Pseudotruncus," pulmonary arterial supply from major aortopulmonary collaterals arteries, arising from descending aorta – controversial entity, misnomer for pulmonary atresia with VSD
- Many variations exist, involving interruption of the aortic arch, absence of a branch pulmonary artery (hemitruncus) and patent ductus arteriosus

Clinical Issues
Presentation
- Progressive congestive heart failure with drop in pulmonary vascular resistance in young infant
- Increasing cyanosis due to shunt reversal with development of pulmonary hypertension

Natural History
- Intractable congestive heart failure
- Eventual shunt reversal with progressive cyanosis and sudden death

Treatment
- Palliative: Banding of main pulmonary artery
- Surgical repair, with placement of conduit between right ventricle and pulmonary artery, and closure of VSD

Prognosis
- Determined by function of pulmonary artery conduit
- Determined by morbidity of conduit replacement

Selected References
1. Rajasinghe HA et al: Long-term follow-up of truncus arteriosus repaired in infancy: A twenty-year experience. J Thorac Cardiovasc Surg 113:869-78, 1997
2. Donnelly LF et al: MR imaging of cono-truncal abnormalities. Am J Roengenol 166:925-8, 1996
3. Chrispin A et al: Transectional echo planar imaging of the heart in cyanotic congenital heart disease. Pediatr Radiol 16:293-7, 1986

Pulmonary Atresia

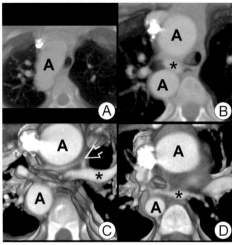

(A-D) Consecutive axial thick slab reconstructions of CT angiogram in 11-year-old cyanotic boy, which demonstrate right aortic arch (A), multiple APCAs originating from descending aorta (asterisks) and confluence of hypoplastic branch pulmonary arteries (arrow in C). Note asymmetry and irregularity of pulmonary vascularity.

Key Facts
- Synonyms: Truncus arteriosus Type 4 = pseudotruncus (misnomer)
- Definition: Absent development of the right ventricular outflow tract (RVOT) and pulmonary valve
- Associated features: Subaortic ventricular septal defect, multiple aorticopulmonary arteries (MAPCAs)
- Classic plain film appearance: "Boot-shaped" heart, right arch, diminutive hilar shadows and irregular pattern of pulmonary vascularity
- Category: Cyanotic, cardiomegaly, irregular pulmonary vasculature
- Hemodynamics
  - Extreme outflow obstruction of right ventricle, (almost) entire cardiac output goes into dilated overriding ascending aorta
  - Balance between flow through pulmonary arteries (PAs, via ductus arteriosus) and MAPCAs determines pulmonary perfusion
  - Pulmonary atresia is at the extreme of the tetralogy of Fallot spectrum

Imaging Findings
General Features
- Best imaging clue: Atresia of right ventricular outflow tract (RVOT)
Chest Radiography Findings
- Extreme "boot-shaped" appearance of the heart
- Right-sided aortic arch common
- Small hilar shadows
- Irregular branching patterns of MAPCAs
Echocardiography Findings
- Characterizes intracardiac anatomy, VSD
- Aortic root override
- Development of branch PAs, their confluence
CT Angiography Findings
- Better than echocardiography for PA anatomy

Pulmonary Atresia

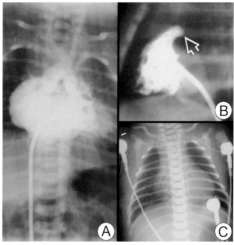

Pulmonary atresia with intact ventricular septum. (A,B) RV injection study shows occlusion at the pulmonary valve (arrow in B). There is an obligatory R → L shunt via patent foramen ovale. (C) Chest radiograph after right Blalock-Taussig shunt placement (note rib splaying) reveals right cardiomegaly and pulmonary oligemia.

- Can be used as road-map for subsequent catheterization

Cardiac Catheterization with Angiography Findings
- Required for selective injection studies of all MAPCAs, true PAs, pressure recordings
- Pulmonary venous wedge injections for retrograde filling of diminutive PAs

MR Findings
- Cardiac-gated T1WI: PAs best seen in long axis images
- Cine-MRI: Helpful for functional cardiac assessment, tricuspid regurgitation
- Gadolinium-MRA for global pulmonary arterial anatomy

Imaging Recommendations
- Initial diagnosis with echocardiography
- CT or MR for assessment of pulmonary arterial anatomy; postoperatively for assessment of shunt/conduit patency
- Cardiac catheterization for hemodynamic assessment, selective injection studies and catheter-based interventions (balloon angioplasty with stenting of peripheral PA stenoses, coil embolization of MAPCAs)

Differential Diagnosis

Tetralogy of Fallot
- At least partial patency of RVOT

Pulmonary Atresia with Intact Ventricular Septum
- Distinct entity from pulmonary atresia with VSD and MAPCAs
- Severe right-sided obstruction → cyanosis, tricuspid regurgitation
- Massively dilated right atrium, small trabeculated right ventricle

Pathology

General
- General path comments

Pulmonary Atresia

- o Constitutes the extreme of the spectrum of RVOT-obstructive (Fallot-type) heart lesions, with complex and highly variable PA anatomy
- Embryology
  - o RVOT obstruction is primary event → hypoplasia of PAs
  - o Persistence or hypertrophy of primitive arterial connections to lungs
  - o Hypertrophy of bronchial arteries
- Pathophysiology
  - o Pulmonary perfusion via ductus arteriosus, MAPCAs
  - o Cyanosis determined by admixture and amount of pulmonary flow
  - o Large amount of pulmonary blood flow → congestive heart failure
- Epidemiology
  - o Rare congenital cyanotic heart lesion, classified together with Fallot

Gross Pathologic, Surgical Features
- Hilar arteries = true PAs
- Presence and confluence of true PAs important for surgical repair
- MAPCAs originating from
  - o Ascending aorta
  - o Brachiocephalic or intercostal arteries
  - o Ductus arteriosus
  - o Descending aorta (most common)

Microscopic Features
- Pulmonary vascular disease develops in vascular bed of high-flow MAPCAs
  - o Increase in cyanosis

Clinical Issues

Presentation
- Progressive cyanosis after birth with closure of ductus arteriosus
- Congestive heart failure with large unobstructed high-flow MAPCAs

Natural History
- Progressive cyanosis due to development of pulmonary vascular disease

Treatment
- Prostaglandin E_1 to keep ductus arteriosus open
- Palliative systemic-to-PA shunt (Blalock-Taussig, central)
- Initial banding of high-flow MAPCAs
- Unifocalization of MAPCAs to true PAs (if existent), to allow for PA growth
- Complete repair with incorporation of MAPCAs and PAs in conduit, RVOT reconstruction, closure of VSD
- Catheter-based interventions (angioplasty of stenoses, embolization of superfluous or bleeding MAPCAs)

Prognosis
- Life expectancy when untreated less than 10 years
- Guarded, depends on feasibility of surgical repair
- Complications from multiple repairs and other interventions

Selected References
1. Powell AJ et al: Accuracy of MRI in evaluation of pulmonary blood supply in patients with complex pulmonary stenosis or atresia. Int J Card Imaging 16:169-74, 2000
2. Westra SJ et al: Cardiac electron-beam CT in children undergoing surgical repair for pulmonary atresia. Radiology 213:502-12, 1999
3. Ichida F et al: Evaluation of pulmonary blood supply by multiplanar cine magnetic resonance imaging in patients with pulmonary atresia and severe pulmonary stenosis. Int J Card Imaging 15:473-81, 1999

Total Anomalous Pulmonary Venous Return

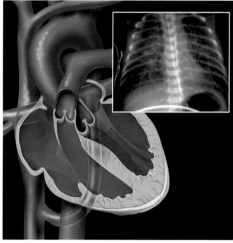

Total anomalous pulmonary venous return (TAPVR) Type III. Drawing illustrates infradiaphragmatic TAPVR to inferior vena cava, constituting obligatory extracardiac L → R shunt. Mixed blood flows to left atrium through patent foramen ovale. Insert: Chest radiograph shows normal heart size and pulmonary edema.

Key Facts
- TAPVR = Total anomalous pulmonary venous return
- Synonym: Total anomalous pulmonary venous return (TAPVR)
- Definition: Failure of connection between pulmonary veins and left atrium
- Three types
  - Supracardiac TAPVR (Type I): "Vertical" common pulmonary vein joins L innominate vein
  - Cardiac TAPVR (Type II): Common pulmonary vein joins coronary sinus
  - Infracardiac TAPVR (Type III): Common pulmonary vein joins portal vein, ductus venosus or inferior vena cava
- Classic plain film appearance
  - Type I: "Snowman" heart
  - Type II: Indistinguishable from atrial septal defect (ASD)
  - Type III: Small heart, reticular pattern in the lungs: Edema
- Category: Cyanotic; heart size and pulmonary vascularity depend on type
- Hemodynamics
  - All pulmonary venous return to R heart (extracardiac L → R shunt)
  - Intracardiac R → L shunt through patent foramen ovale (PFO)
  - All types are admixture lesions

Imaging Findings
General Features
- Best imaging clue: No pulmonary veins connecting to left atrium
Chest Radiography Findings
- Cardiomegaly (Types I and II), small heart (Type III)
- Shunt vascularity (Types I and II), pulmonary edema (Type III)
- Wide mediastinum (Type I, "snowman heart"), narrow mediastinum (Types II and III, thymic atrophy)
- Left vertical vein often visible in Type I

Total Anomalous Pulmonary Venous Return

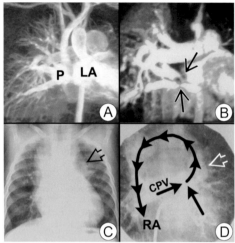

TAPVR III after repair. (A, B) Gd-MRA shows anastomotic stenoses (arrows in B) between pulmonary veins & pericardial patch (P) to left atrium (LA) conduit. TAPVR I. (C) Chest radiograph: "Snowman" heart with vertical vein (arrow). (D) Venous angiogram: Flow direction from common pulmonary vein (CPV) to R atrium.

Echocardiography Findings
- Lack of connection of pulmonary veins to left atrium
- Right-sided chamber enlargement in Types I and II
- PFO
- Associated cardiac and abdominal situs abnormalities
- Limited for assessment of postoperative venous obstruction

CT Findings
- 3D CT angiography: For pre- and postoperative pulmonary vein caliber
- Thickened interlobular septa, peribronchial cuffing and ground-glass opacities suggest postoperative anastomotic pulmonary venous stenosis

MR Findings
- Cardiac-gated T1WI: Anomalous connection best seen in axial plane
- Cine-MRI: For functional cardiac assessment, flow jets, regurgitation
- Phase-contrast MRA: For detection of pulmonary vein anastomotic stenosis (flow velocities > 100 cm/sec are diagnostic)

Angiography Findings
- Seldom required for primary diagnosis
- After repair: For diagnosis and treatment of anastomotic pulmonary venous stenosis

Imaging Recommendations
- Primary diagnosis with echocardiography
- CT, MRI for postoperative pulmonary vein anastomotic stenosis

Differential Diagnosis

Cor Triatriatum
- Pulmonary venous connection occurred but remains stenotic

Hypoplastic Left Heart Syndrome

Persistent Fetal Circulation Syndrome, Primary Pulmonary Hypertension
- Associated with severe hyaline membrane disease, meconium aspiration

Total Anomalous Pulmonary Venous Return

Pathology

<u>General</u>
- General path comments
  - All pulmonary veins eventually drain into right atrium
  - Low systemic blood flow may lead to associated hypoplasia of left-sided cardiac chambers
- Genetics
  - No specific genetic defect found
  - Occasionally associated with other complex cyanotic heart disease, asplenia syndrome, atrioventricular canal
- Embryology
  - Lack of normal incorporation of primitive common pulmonary vein into posterior wall of left atrium
  - Persistence and enlargement of embryological pathways for pulmonary venous return via umbilicovitelline and cardinal veins
- Pathophysiology
  - All types have PFO to allow for obligatory R → L flow, leading to varying degrees of cyanosis (less severe in Types I, II: Pulmonary hypercirculation)
  - Non-obstructive TAPVR (Types I and II): ASD physiology, pulmonary plethora, congestive heart failure
  - Obstructive TAPVR (Type III): Common pulmonary vein is obstructed by diaphragmatic hiatus → pulmonary venous congestion and edema
- Epidemiology
  - 1-3% of congenital heart disease, More frequent in neonatal period

<u>Gross Pathologic, Surgical Features</u>
- Common pulmonary vein is anastomosed via window with left atrium, and all other abnormal pulmonary venous connections are ligated

Clinical Issues

<u>Presentation</u>
- Types I, II: Initially asymptomatic, followed by congestive heart failure
- Type III: Severe cyanosis at birth
- Patent ductus arteriosus: Persistent fetal circulation

<u>Natural History</u>
- No patients survive without surgical treatment

<u>Treatment</u>
- Prostaglandin E_1 to improve systemic perfusion in pulmonary hypertension
- Early surgical anastomosis of pulmonary venous confluence to left atrium

<u>Prognosis: Highly Variable</u>
- Type I, II: Initially asymptomatic, with gradual development of congestive heart failure (ASD physiology)
- Type III, obstructive forms: Death within a month
- After surgical repair: Determined by associated cardiac anomalies and development of pulmonary vein anastomotic stenosis

Selected References
1. Videlefsky N et al: Magnetic resonance phase-shift velocity mapping in pediatric patients with pulmonary venous obstruction. Am J Cardiol 87:589-93, 2001
2. Chen SJ et al: Validation of pulmonary venous obstruction by electron beam tomography in children with congenital heart disease. Ann Thor Surg 71:1690-2, 2001
3. Kim TH et al: Helical CT angiography and three-dimensional reconstruction of total anomalous pulmonary venous connections in neonates and infants. Am J Roentgenol 175:1381-6, 2000

Scimitar Syndrome

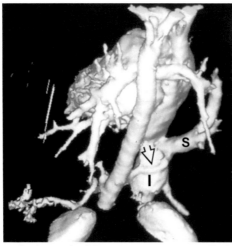

Posterior view of surface rendered CT angiogram in seven-year-old girl with scimitar syndrome, who presented with recurrent right lung infections, shows total venous drainage of right lung via scimitar vein (S) to inferior vena cava (I), and systemic artery (arrow) from celiac axis to right lung base.

Key Facts
- Synonyms: Hypogenetic lung syndrome, congenital venolobar syndrome
- Definition: Right lung hypoplasia, anomalous right pulmonary venous connection to inferior vena cava (IVC)
- Often associated: Anomalous systemic arterial supply to right lung base
- Classic plain film appearance: Right lung hypoplasia, dextroversion of the heart, scimitar vein in right medial costophrenic sulcus
- Category: Acyanotic, partial anomalous pulmonary venous return (PAPVR)
- Hemodynamics: Venous flow from right lung returns into right atrium → volume overload of right heart (ASD physiology)

Imaging Findings
General Features
- Best imaging clue: Scimitar sign = curved anomalous venous trunk, resembling a Turkish sword, in right medial costophrenic sulcus near right heart border, that increases in caliber in a caudad direction
Chest Radiography Findings
- Right lung hypoplasia
- Dextroversion of heart (no dextrocardia: Apex is directed toward left)
- Prominent right atrium, active pulmonary vascular congestion: Shunt vascularity
- Scimitar vein
Echocardiography Findings
- No right pulmonary veins entering left atrium
- Scimitar vein connecting to IVC
Angiography Findings
- Scimitar vein opacifies during venous phase of pulmonary artery injection
- Injection of abdominal aorta: Anomalous systemic arterial supply to right lung base (originating from celiac axis, right phrenic artery, descending aorta)

Scimitar Syndrome

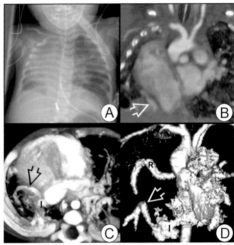

Scimitar syndrome in infant with pulmonary hypertension. (A) Chest radiograph shows right lung hypoplasia. (B,C,D) 3D reconstructions of CT angiogram demonstrate right heart dilatation, scimitar vein (arrow) to inferior vena cava (I) and prominent right pulmonary artery (R), despite ipsilateral lung hypoplasia.

- Used for coil embolization of systemic artery

CT Findings
- Axial images show scimitar vein joining IVC
- CT angiography with three-dimensional (3D) reconstruction most helpful to demonstrate anomalous systemic arterial supply, right pulmonary and mainstem bronchus hypoplasia

MR Findings
- Cardiac-gated T1WI: Anomalous pulmonary venous connection best seen in axial and coronal planes
- Phase-contrast MRA for shunt flow calculation
- Gadolinium-MRA, coronal acquisition with 3D reconstruction for anomalous right pulmonary venous and arterial development

Imaging Recommendations
- CTA or MRA are better than echocardiography for complete assessment, and can replace diagnostic angiocardiography
- Angiography reserved for coil embolization

Differential Diagnosis

Other Forms of Partial Anomalous Pulmonary Venous Connection
- Right pulmonary vein(s) to azygous vein, superior vena cava, right atrium (with sinus venosus atrial septal defect)

True Dextrocardia with Abdominal Situs Solitus
- Other complex cardiac anomalies

Isolated Right Pulmonary Hypoplasia
- Normal right pulmonary venous connection to left atrium

Pulmonary Sequestration
- Mass in right lung base not connected to bronchial tree, with systemic arterial supply and venous drainage to pulmonary (intralobar) or systemic (extralobar) veins

Scimitar Syndrome

Pathology

<u>General</u>
- General path comments
  - Associated in 25% with other anomalies
    - Atrial septal defect most common
    - Ventricular septal defect, tetralogy of Fallot, patent ductus arteriosus
    - Diaphragmatic abnormalities: Accessory hemidiaphragm, hernia
- Genetics
  - No specific genetic defect identified
- Embryology
  - Primary abnormality in development of right lung, with secondary anomalous pulmonary venous connection
- Pathophysiology
  - Obligatory left to right shunt to right atrium: ASD physiology

<u>Gross Pathologic, Surgical Features</u>
- Right lung (including pulmonary arterial and bronchial) hypoplasia
- Anomalous right pulmonary venous drainage to IVC (most frequent) or right atrium, superior vena cava, azygous vein, portal vein, hepatic vein

<u>Microscopic Features</u>
- Normal right lung parenchyma (as opposed to sequestration)
- Systemic artery branches anastomose with right pulmonary artery vascular bed in right lung base
- Long-standing shunt: Pulmonary vascular disease, leading to irreversible pulmonary hypertension (Eisenmenger)

Clinical Issues

<u>Presentation: Depending on Size of Left to Right Shunt</u>
- Newborn: Congestive heart failure, right heart volume overload, pulmonary hypertension
- Young child: Recurrent infections in right lung base
- Older child: Often asymptomatic (incidental finding on chest radiograph)

<u>Natural History</u>
- Large shunt: Development of irreversible pulmonary hypertension

<u>Treatment</u>
- Embolization of systemic arterial supply
- Baffling of common right pulmonary vein onto left atrium

<u>Prognosis</u>
- Moderate to poor with neonatal presentation
- May be asymptomatic for many years with small shunt

Selected References
1. Huddleston CB et al: Scimitar syndrome presenting in infancy. Ann Thor Surg 67:154-60, 1999
2. Vrachliotis TG et al: Hypogenetic lung syndrome: Functional and anatomic evaluation with magnetic resonance imaging and magnetic resonance angiography. J Magn Reson Imaging 6:798-800, 1996
3. Woodring JH et al: Congenital venolobar syndrome revisited. Radiographics 14:349-69, 1994

Hypoplastic Left Heart Syndrome

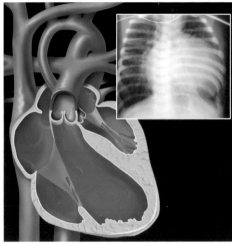

Hypoplastic left heart syndrome. Drawing depicts hypoplasia of left atrium, left ventricle, aortic valve and ascending aorta. Systemic flow depends on patency of ductus arteriosus. Oxygenation occurs by flow admixture in right atrium, with L → R shunting through foramen ovale. Insert: Typical chest radiograph in neonate.

Key Facts
- Synonyms: Aortic atresia
- Definition: Hypoplasia/atresia of the ascending aorta, aortic valve, left ventricle and mitral valve
- Secondary findings: Patent ductus arteriosus, juxtaductal coarctation
- Most severe congenital heart lesion presenting in neonatal period, with congestive heart failure, cardiogenic shock and cyanosis
- Classic imaging appearance: Retrograde flow in hypoplastic ascending aorta for head, neck and coronary perfusion
- Category: Cyanotic, cardiomegaly, increased pulmonary vascularity
- Hemodynamics
  - Severe obstruction to flow in systemic circulation (= ductus-dependent)
  - Volume overload in pulmonary circulation
  - Left-to-right shunting through foramen ovale
  - Flow admixture in right atrium → severe cyanosis

Imaging Findings
General Features
- Best imaging clue: Hypoplasia of ascending aorta, left ventricle
Chest Radiography Findings
- Cardiomegaly
- Pulmonary venous congestion with interstitial fluid
- Hyperinflation
- Narrow mediastinum due to thymic atrophy
Echocardiography Findings
- Diminutive ascending aorta < 5 mm
- Small, thick-walled left ventricle
- Dilatation of right-sided cardiac chambers and pulmonary artery
- Patent ductus arteriosus, left-to-right shunting through foramen ovale

Hypoplastic Left Heart Syndrome

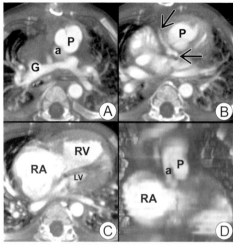

Norwood repair for HLHS. Axial slab (A-C) and coronal (D) reformats of CT angiogram show hypoplastic ascending aorta (a) perfusing the coronaries (arrows), large main pulmonary artery (P) serving as a cardiac output conduit, right cavopulmonary (Glenn, G) shunt and relative cardiac chamber size (RA, RV, LV).

Cardiac Catheterization with Angiography Findings
- Aortography can be done via umbilical artery catheter
  - Retrograde flow in hypoplastic ascending aorta
  - Some filling of pulmonary arteries via ductus arteriosus

CT, MR Findings
- Occasionally performed after staged Norwood procedure
- Patency of aortopulmonary (Blalock-Taussig) and cavopulmonary (Glenn) shunts, pulmonary artery anatomy
- Functional assessment of univentricular heart with cine MRI, prior to Fontan operation

Imaging Recommendations
- Primary diagnosis made with echocardiography in majority of cases
- Postoperative: Functional MRI and interventional catheterizations for residua/sequelae of Fontan operation

Differential Diagnosis: Congestive Heart Failure in Newborn
Critical Aortic Atenosis, Infantile Coarctation, Interrupted Aortic Arch
- Pressure overload of normally-developed left ventricle

Cranial (Vein of Galen) or Hepatic Arteriovenous Malformation
- Structurally normal heart with volume overload of all chambers

Cardiomyopathy, Endocardial Fibroelastosis
- Globally enlarged, structurally normal heart, myocardial dysfunction

Coronary Arteriovenous Fistula
- Right coronary originates from pulmonary artery, myocardial infarction

Severe Arrhythmias – Paroxysmal Supraventricular Tachycardia
- Characteristic electrocardiogram

Hypoplastic Left Heart Syndrome

Pathology
<u>General</u>
- Underdevelopment of left-sided cardiac structures
- Compatible with normal fetal hemodynamics → no fetal compromise
- Genetics: No clear genetic defect demonstrated in majority of cases
- Embryology
  - Abnormal partitioning of primitive conotruncus into left and right ventricular outflow tracts → hypoplasia/atresia of aortic valve
  - Diminished prenatal antegrade flow through aorta → underdevelopment of left ventricle and ascending aorta
- Pathophysiology
  - Severe obstruction to outflow of left ventricle, which is diminutive
  - Pulmonary venous flow shunts through foramen ovale into right atrium
  - Dilated right cardiac chambers and pulmonary artery
  - Systemic perfusion via patent ductus arteriosus
- Epidemiology
  - 1-3 per 10,000 live births, M:F = 2:1
  - Fourth most common congenital heart lesion presenting under 1 year

<u>Gross Pathologic, Surgical Features</u>
- Severe hypoplasia of left-sided cardiac chambers and ascending aorta
- Endocardial fibroelastosis in small, thick-walled left ventricle

Clinical Issues
<u>Presentation</u>
- No circulatory symptoms immediately at birth but rapid deterioration
- Congestive heart failure (volume overload pulmonary circulation)
- Cardiogenic shock after closure of ductus arteriosus
- Cyanosis (flow admixture in right heart)

<u>Natural History</u>
- Death within days/weeks when untreated

<u>Treatment</u>
- Medical: Prostaglandin E_1 to keep ductus arteriosus open
- Emergency Rashkind balloon atrial septostomy in case of flow restriction across atrial septal defect
- Palliative repair
  - Norwood: Construction of neo-aorta from pulmonary artery, atrial septectomy, Blalock-Taussig shunt for pulmonary perfusion (3 weeks)
  - Conversion to hemi-Fontan (Glenn shunt between superior vena cava and right pulmonary artery, 4-6 month)
  - Fontan: Fenestrated venous conduit through right atrium of inferior caval flow to right pulmonary artery (1.5-2 year)
- In some centers: Cardiac transplantation

<u>Prognosis</u>
- Poor without treatment; has improved substantially in recent years
- Determined by complications, residua and sequelae of staged Norwood repair and Fontan operation (right ventricular dysfunction, venous hypertension)

Selected References
1.   Bardo DM et al: Hypoplastic left heart syndrome. Radiographics 21:705-17, 2001
2.   Norwood WI: Hypoplastic left heart syndrome. Ann Thorac Surgery 688-95, 1991
3.   Kondo C et al: Nuclear magnetic resonance imaging of the palliative operation for hypoplastic left heart syndrome. J Am Coll Cardiol 18:817-23, 1991

Heterotaxia Syndrome

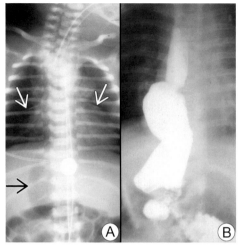

Asplenia syndrome. (A) Chest radiograph in severely cyanotic neonate shows levocardia and right-sided stomach bubble (black arrow), midline liver shadow and bilateral minor fissures (white arrows), indicating tri-lobed lungs (bilateral right-sidedness). (B) Barium study depicts gastric malposition and malrotation.

Key Facts
- Synonyms: Situs ambiguus, cardiosplenic syndromes, Ivemark syndrome
- Definition: Disturbance of the normal left-right asymmetry in the position of thoracic and abdominal organs
- Classic plain film appearance: Transverse midline liver, discrepancy between position of cardiac apex and stomach, bilateral left- or right-sidedness in the chest, findings of congenital heart disease (CHD)
- Two major subtypes
  - o Asplenia syndrome = double right-sidedness
    - Absence of a spleen
    - Inferior vena cava (IVC) and aorta on same side of spine
    - Bilateral superior vena cavae (SVC)
    - Right isomerism of atrial appendages
    - Bilateral tri-lobed lungs
    - Bilaterally symmetrical steep (right-sided) eparterial bronchi
    - Associated with severe cyanotic CHD (atrioventricular septal defect, common atrioventricular valve, double outlet right ventricle, transposition, pulmonary stenosis/atresia)
    - Abnormalities of pulmonary venous connections: Total anomalous pulmonary venous return – often obstructed, below diaphragm
  - o Polysplenia syndrome = double left-sidedness
    - Multiple spleens
    - Dilated azygous vein, no infrahepatic IVC, hepatic veins drain separately into common atrium
    - Bilateral SVC
    - Left isomerism of atrial appendages
    - Bilateral bi-lobed lungs
    - Bilaterally symmetrical horizontal (left-sided) hyparterial bronchi
    - Associated with less severe CHD (common atrium, ventricular septal defect (VSD))

Heterotaxia Syndrome

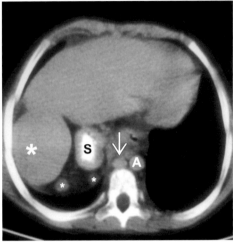

Polysplenia syndrome. CT section through lower chest and upper abdomen shows levocardia, right-sided stomach (S), multiple spleens (*) and prominent azygos vein (arrow) to the right of aorta (A), indicative of azygos continuation of inferior vena cava.

- Abnormalities of systemic venous connections: Azygos continuation of inferior vena cava

Imaging Findings

General Features
- Best imaging clue: Abnormal symmetry in chest and abdomen

Chest Radiography Findings
- Asplenia syndrome
  - Bilateral minor fissures
  - Symmetrical main stem bronchi with narrow carinal angle
  - Cardiomegaly, pulmonary edema
- Polysplenia syndrome
  - No minor fissure on either side
  - Symmetrical main stem bronchi with wide carinal angle
  - Absent IVC shadow on lateral film, prominent azygos shadow on AP
- Both syndromes
  - Transverse liver
  - Right-sided stomach bubble with levocardia, left-sided stomach bubble with dextrocardia, or midline stomach

Echocardiography Findings
- Often definitive test for characterization of intracardiac anomalies, abnormal systemic and/or pulmonary venous connections, segmental description of atrioventricular and ventriculoarterial relationships

CT, MR Findings
- Multiplanar imaging (coronal, axial) of chest and upper abdomen for demonstration of situs abnormalities, systemic and pulmonary venous connections, segmental analysis of intracardiac connections and defects
- Allows for complete preoperative diagnosis of all relevant abnormalities

Heterotaxia Syndrome

Other Modality Findings
- Upper GI study: Malrotation is frequently associated

Imaging Recommendations
- Echocardiography, followed by MRI

Differential Diagnosis

Situs Inversus Totalis
- Mirror image of normal
- Low association with CHD; may be associated with immobile cilia syndrome (Kartagener's): Sinusitis, bronchiectasis, infertility

Dextroversion of the Heart
- Heart is positioned in right chest with apex and stomach still directed toward the left
- In right pulmonary hypoplasia (scimitar syndrome), left-sided mass lesions (diaphragmatic hernia, cystic adenomatoid malformation of lung)

Pathology

General
- General path comments
  - Heterotaxy syndrome represents a spectrum, with overlap between classic asplenia and polysplenia manifestations, and other anomalies
- Genetics
  - No specific genetic defect in majority (usually sporadic)
- Embryology
  - Early embryological disturbance, leading to complex anomalies
- Pathophysiology
  - Determined by complexity of associated CHD
- Epidemiology
  - Prevalence 1 per 22,000 to 24,000; 1-3% of CHD
  - Asplenia is more common in boys; equal sex ratio for polysplenia

Clinical Issues

Presentation
- Asplenia: Male neonate with severe cyanosis, susceptibility for infections
- Polysplenia: More variable, may present later in life
- Heterotaxia syndromes may be associated with malrotation, volvulus, absent gallbladder, extrahepatic biliary atresia

Natural History, Prognosis
- Mortality in 1st year: 85% in asplenia, 65% in polysplenia

Treatment
- Supportive, prostaglandins, antibiotic prophylaxis (asplenia)
- Early biventricular repair if possible
- Univentricular repair: Conversion to Fontan operation
- Polysplenia: Anastomosis of azygos vein to pulmonary artery (Kawashima operation)

Selected References
1. Hong YK et al: Efficacy of MRI in complicated congenital heart disease with visceral heterotaxy syndrome. J Comput Assist Tomogr 24:671-82, 2000
2. Applegate KE et al: Situs revisited: Imaging of heterotaxy syndrome. RadioGraphics 19:837-52, 1999
3. Geva T et al: Role of spin echo and cine magnetic resonance imaging in presurgical planning of heterotaxy syndrome. Circulation 90:348-56, 1994

Septal Defects (ASD, VSD)

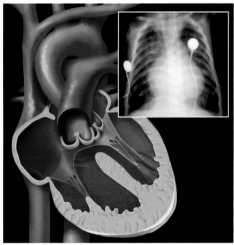

Septal defects. Drawing illustrates complete atrioventricular septal defect (AVSD): Low (septum primum) ASD, high (inlet perimembranous) VSD, straddling common AV valve, enlarged pulmonary artery. Insert: Chest radiograph in Down's baby with AVSD: Right-sided cardiomegaly, shunt vascularity and hyperinflation.

Key Facts
- Definition: Cardiac anomalies characterized by one or more defects in the septa dividing the right-sided from the left-sided cardiac chambers
- Classic plain film appearance: Cardiomegaly, convex pulmonary artery segment, active pulmonary vascular congestion = shunt vascularity
- Category: Acyanotic, cardiomegaly, increased pulmonary vascularity
- Main groups
  - Atrial septal defect (ASD)
    - Septum primum defect
    - Septum secundum defect
    - Patent foramen ovale
    - Sinus venosus defect
  - Ventricular septal defect (VSD)
    - Inlet septal defect
    - Muscular = trabecular septal defect
    - Outlet septal defect
    - Perimembranous septal defect (75%)
  - Atrioventricular septal defect (AVSD)
    - Synonyms: Atrioventricular canal, endocardial cushion defect
    - Ostium primum ASD
    - Inlet perimembranous VSD
    - "Cleft" mitral valve
    - Incomplete or complete AVSD, straddling valve leaflets
- Hemodynamics: Volume overload leading to enlargement of receiving cardiac segment (and all segments distally to that)
  - ASD: Right atrium, **not** left atrium; small aorta
  - VSD: Right ventricle and left atrium; small aorta
  - ASVD: Right atrium and ventricle, **not** left atrium; small aorta

Septal Defects (ASD, VSD)

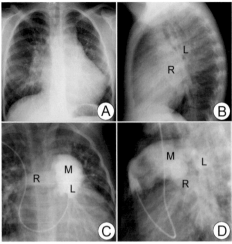

Pulmonary hypertension in patient with untreated VSD, PDA and new-onset cyanosis. (A,B) Chest radiographs show right ventricular prominence and central dilatation of main pulmonary artery (M), right (R) and left (L) pulmonary arteries (PAs). (C,D) Correlative pulmonary angiogram, note "pruned" appearance of PAs.

Imaging Findings

General Features
- Specific chamber enlargement, dependent on location of shunt
- All intracardiac shunt lesions have small aorta

Chest Radiography Findings
- Cardiomegaly
- Convex pulmonary artery segment, increased ("shunt") vascularity
- Interstitial fluid with congestive heart failure
- Hyperinflation due to bronchial compression by dilated pulmonary arteries

Echocardiography Findings
- Characterizes type, location and number of septal defect(s)
- Specific chamber enlargement
- Associated valvular dysfunction

MR Findings
- Cardiac-gated T1WI: Septal defects best seen on long axis images
- Cine-MRI: For functional cardiac assessment, flow jets, regurgitation

Cardiac Catheterization and Angiography Findings
- Seldom required for primary diagnosis
- Used for ASD closure with Amplatz device

Imaging Recommendations
- Primary diagnosis with echocardiography
- Catheterization is needed when pulmonary hypertension is suspected

Differential Diagnosis

Patent Ductus Arteriosus: Large aorta

High-Output Conditions: Global Cardiomegaly, Wide Vascular Pedicle
- Extracardiac arteriovenous malformation, e.g. vein of Galen
- Anemias

Septal Defects (ASD, VSD)

Myocardial Dysfunction: Global Cardiomegaly, Narrow Vascular Pedicle
- Cardiomyopathies
- Arrhythmias

Pericardial Effusion: "Water Bottle" - Shaped Heart Shadow

Pathology
General
- General path comments
  - Location of VSD important for surgical repair
  - Multiple defects occur, especially in the trabecular septum
- Genetics
  - No specific genetic defect in majority
  - AVSD associated with trisomy 21 (Down syndrome)
- Embryology
  - Complex, dependent on location of defect and associated anomalies
- Pathophysiology
  - Volume overload to pulmonary circulation
  - ASD: Low pressure shunt
  - VSD, AVSD: High pressure shunts
  - Eventually all lead to pulmonary hypertension
- Epidemiology
  - Most common congenital cardiac lesions
  - True incidence of septal defects > reported (many close spontaneously)

Clinical Issues
Presentation: Dependent on Systemic/Pulmonary Pressures
- Age at presentation: AVSD < VSD < ASD
- Congestive heart failure without cyanosis

Natural History
- Most small muscular VSDs close spontaneously
- Untreated large shunt: Development of pulmonary vascular disease = Eisenmenger's reaction: Irreversible pulmonary hypertension
- Reversal of shunt from right to left: Late onset cyanosis

Treatment
- Surgical closure of shunt lesion
- Temporizing procedure: Pulmonary artery banding
- Percutaneous closure with device is possible for ASD

Prognosis
- Isolated septal defects: Excellent prognosis after closure
- Many muscular VSDs close spontaneously
- Associated cardiac anomalies determine final outcome
- Untreated with pulmonary hypertension: Shunt reversal, risk for paradoxical embolus to brain, stroke and abscess
- Lifetime risk of bacterial endocarditis

Selected References
1.   Brenner LD et al: Quantification of left to right atrial shunts with velocity-encoded cine nuclear magnetic resonance imaging. J Am Coll Cardiol 1992:1246-50, 1992
2.   Parsons JM et al: Morphological evaluation of atrioventricular septal defects by magnetic resonance imaging. Br Heart J 64:138-45, 1990
3.   Baker EJ etal: Magnetic resonance imaging at a high field strength of ventricular septal defects in infants. Br Heart J 62:305-10, 1989

Patent Ductus Arteriosus

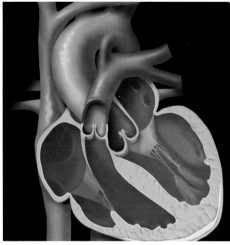

Patent ductus arteriosus (PDA). Drawing depicts ductus, resulting in L → R shunt. Note dilated left atrium and ventricle.

Key Facts
- Synonyms: PDA, persistent arterial duct, patent ductus Botalli
- Definition: Persistent postnatal patency of the normal prenatal connection from the pulmonary artery to the proximal descending aorta
- Classic plain film appearance: Cardiomegaly (left atrium and ventricle), increased pulmonary flow, large aortic arch with "ductus bump"
- Category: Acyanotic, increased pulmonary flow
- Hemodynamics: L → R shunt between aorta and pulmonary artery
- PDA is frequently an essential part of complex congenital heart disease
  - Hypoplastic left heart syndrome, preductal coarctation, interrupted aortic arch: Conduit for systemic perfusion (R → L flow)
  - D-transposition: Necessary admixture between pulmonary and systemic circuits (L → R flow)
  - Pulmonary atresia and other severe cyanotic heart disease: Conduit for pulmonary perfusion (L → R flow)
- PDA is part of persistent fetal circulation syndrome (severe lung disease-meconium aspiration, primary pulmonary hypertension): R → L flow

Imaging Findings
General Features
- Best imaging clue: Ductus bump
Chest Radiography Findings
- Cardiomegaly: Left atrium, left ventricle
- Increased pulmonary flow
- Wide vascular pedicle (ascending aorta, ductus bump)
Echocardiography Findings
- M-mode: Increased left atrium to aorta ratio
- Suprasternal notch view: Direct visualization of ductus
- Doppler
  - For flow direction through ductus

Patent Ductus Arteriosus

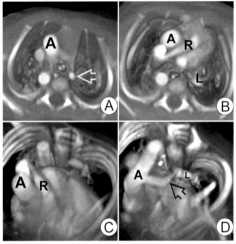

Patent ductus arteriosus in newborn with complex cyanotic anomaly. (A-D) 3D rendered CT angiogram shows right aortic arch (A), isolated right (R) branch pulmonary artery (PA), absent central left branch PA, with peripheral left (L) PA supplied via left ductus arteriosus (arrows), originating from left subclavian artery.

  o Diastolic flow reversal in descending and abdominal aorta

<u>CT Findings</u>
- CT angiography with volume rendition of aortic arch depicts ductus

<u>MR Findings</u>
- Cardiac-gated T1WI, cine gradient echo
  - o Sagittal-oblique plane through aortic arch depicts ductus
- 3D gadolinium MRA with volume rendition

<u>Cardiac Catheterization and Angiography Findings</u>
- Only needed for associated complex cyanotic heart disease

<u>Imaging Recommendations</u>
- Treatment based in majority on echocardiographic findings only

Differential Diagnosis

<u>Other Causes of L → R Shunting</u>
- Septal defects, atrioventricular canal

<u>Persistent Fetal Circulation Syndrome</u>
- Pulmonary hypertension (primary or secondary to severe lung disease)
- Patent foramen ovale, PDA secondary to profound irreversible hypoxia

Pathology

<u>General</u>
- General path comments
  - o In normal neonate ductus arteriosus closes functionally 18-24 hours after birth, anatomically at 1 month of age
  - o PDA is persistence of normal prenatal structure after birth
- Etiology-pathogenesis
  - o Persistent postnatal hypoxia → failure of contraction of ductus
  - o Associated with maternal rubella
- Genetics

o No specific genetic defect identified in most cases of isolated PDA
- Embryology
  o Ductus originates from primitive sixth aortic arch
- Pathophysiology (for simple PDA)
  o L → R shunt to pulmonary artery
  o Volume overload of left-sided cardiac cambers
  o With pulmonary hypertension pressure overload of right ventricle
  o Diastolic flow reversal in aorta can lead to renal and intestinal hypoperfusion: Renal dysfunction, necrotizing enterocolitis
- Epidemiology
  o 10-12% of congenital heart disease
  o 1 per 2500-5000 live births
  o Slightly more common in females
  o Associated with prematurity (21-35%)

Gross Pathologic, Surgical Features
- Patent arterial duct, most often wider on aortic side
- Contractile tissue on pulmonary side, spirally arranged muscle bundles
- When closed: Forms ligamentum arteriosum, which may calcify (incidental calcification in aortopulmonary window on chest radiograph or CT)
- Can be right-sided

Clinical Issues

Presentation
- Characteristic machinery-like murmur, bounding peripheral pulses
- Congestive heart failure
- Premature infant recovering from hyaline membrane disease: Shunt though ductus becomes clinically manifest with drop in pulmonary vascular resistance → clinical and radiographic deterioration

Natural History
- Irreversible pulmonary hypertension (Eisenmenger's physiology) resulting in shunt reversal, development of cyanosis

Treatment
- Premature infants: Indomethacin
- To keep ductus open (cyanotic heart disease): Prostaglandin E_1
- Term infants, older children: Surgical clipping or ligation
- Endovascular closure with duct occluder device is now feasible

Prognosis
- Isolated PDA: Excellent with early closure
- When associated with complex heart disease: As determined by underlying disorder
- Persistent fetal circulation, pulmonary hypertension: Treatment with extracorporeal membrane oxygenation (ECMO) is often necessary to disrupt vicious circle

Selected References
1. Schmidt M et al: Magnetic resonance imaging of ductus arteriosus: Botallo apertus in adulthood. In J Cardiol 68:225-9, 1999
2. Sharma S et al: Computed tomography and magnetic resonance findings in long standing ductus. Angiology 47:393-8, 1996
3. Chien CT et al: Potential diagnosis of hemodynamic abnormalities in patent ductus arteriosus by cine magnetic resonance imaging. Am Heart J 122:1065-73, 1991

Ebstein's Anomaly

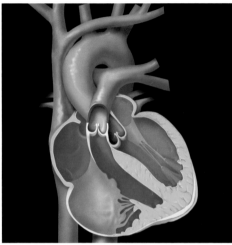

Ebstein's anomaly of the tricuspid valve. Drawing depicts downward displacement of the posterior valve leaflet, which has become incorporated into the right ventricular (RV) wall, leading to "atrialization" of the inflow portion of the RV. Cyanosis results from R → L shunting through patent foramen ovale.

Key Facts
- Definition: Downward displacement of the septal and posterior leaflets of the tricuspid valve
- Classic plain film appearance: Massive right-sided cardiomegaly ("box-shaped" heart)
- Category: Cyanotic, (severe) cardiomegaly, normal or decreased pulmonary vascularity
- Hemodynamics
  - Volume overload to right heart
  - R → L shunting through patent foramen ovale (PFO) → cyanosis

Imaging Findings
General Features
- Best imaging clue: Downward displacement of septal tricuspid leaflet

Chest Radiography Findings
- Severe R-sided cardiomegaly
- Small vascular pedicle
- May mimic large pericardial effusion

Echocardiography Findings
- Right chamber enlargement, "atrialized" portion of right ventricle
- Tricuspid regurgitation
- PFO with R → L shunting

Radionuclide Imaging Finding
- Decreased left ventricular ejection fraction in 50%

Angiography Findings
- Characteristic notch at inferior right ventricular border at insertion of displaced anterior tricuspid leaflet
- Seldom required for primary diagnosis

Ebstein's Anomaly

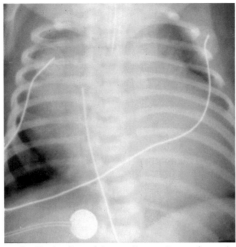

Ebstein's anomaly. Chest radiograph in cyanotic neonate reveals massively enlarged, "box-shaped" heart. Pulmonary vascularity is barely visible. Echocardiography showed characteristic tricuspid valve deformity with severe regurgitation, right-sided chamber enlargement, R → L shunting through PFO.

MR Findings
- Cardiac-gated T1WI: Right chamber best seen on long axis images
- Gradient-echo (GRE) cine-MRI: Helpful for functional cardiac assessment, tricuspid regurgitation

Imaging Recommendations
- Anatomic and functional assessment with echocardiography in infants and cine MRI in (young) adults

Differential Diagnosis

Large Atrial Septal Defect (ASD)
- Non-cyanotic
- Increased pulmonary vascularity
- L → R flow through ASD

Pericardial Effusion
- Acyanotic
- Easy differentiation with echocardiography

Tricuspid Insufficiency
- Primary, due to dysplastic valve
- Often secondary to pulmonary atresia with intact ventricular septum

Uhl's Anomaly and Arrhythmogenic Right Ventricular Dysplasia (ARVD)
- Similar but distinct entities with congenital absence (Uhl's) or fatty infiltration (ARVD) of right ventricular myocardium
- May be differentiated from Ebstein's with spin-echo and cine MRI

Pathology

General
- General path comments
  - Massive right-sided chamber enlargement

- o Three compartments: Right atrium, atrialized non-contracting inlet portion and functional outlet portion of right ventricle
- Genetics
  - o Most often sporadic
- Embryology
  - o Insufficient separation of tricuspid valve leaflets and chordae tendineae from right ventricular endocardium
- Pathophysiology
  - o Massive tricuspid regurgitation
  - o Volume overload to right side of heart
  - o R → L shunt through PFO
  - o Left ventricular diastolic dysfunction may result from massive right-sided cardiac enlargement
  - o Arrhythmias due to conduction abnormalities are common
- Epidemiology
  - o < 1% of congenital cardiac anomalies, incidence 1/210,000 live births
  - o M:F = 1:1

Gross Pathologic, Surgical Features
- Thickened valve leaflets, adherent to underlying myocardium
- Downward displacement of septal and posterior tricuspid leaflets
- Normally placed, redundant "sail-like" anterior tricuspid leaflet
- May occur on left side of the heart with congenitally corrected (L) transposition

Clinical Issues
Presentation
- Spectrum of findings, some patients are asymptomatic
- Hydrops fetalis in severe neonatal cases
- Chronic right heart failure
- Presence of cyanosis depends on balance between right and left atrial pressures

Natural History
- Sudden death due to fatal atrial arrhythmias
- Uncomplicated pregnancies possible in women with hemodynamically well-balanced lesions

Treatment
- Tricuspid valve replacement and/or reconstruction

Prognosis
- Highly variable, dependent on hemodynamic significance of tricuspid regurgitation, presence of cyanosis

Selected References
1. Ammash NM et al: Mimics of Ebstein's anomaly. Am Heart J 134:508-13, 1997
2. Choi YH at al: MR imaging of Ebstein's anomaly of the tricuspid valve. Am J Roentgenol 163:539-43, 1994
3. Kastler B et al: Potential role of MR imaging in the diagnostic management of Ebstein's anomaly in a newborn. J Comput Assist Tomogr 14:825-7, 1990

PocketRadiologist™
Cardiac
Top 100 Diagnoses

VALVULAR

Aortic Stenosis

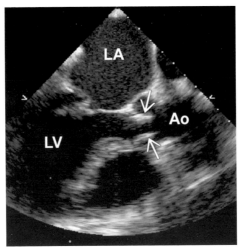

TEE of the aortic valve showing thickened aortic valve leaflets (arrows) with impaired opening of the valve during systole.

Key Facts
- Narrowing of the aortic outflow tract at valvular, supravalvular, or subvalvular levels, causing obstruction to flow from the left ventricle (LV) into the ascending aorta
- Thickening, fusion and/or calcification of the aortic valve apparatus
- High velocity jet of blood ejected into left ventricular outflow during systole
- High peak systolic pressure gradient
- Severe aortic stenosis (AS) leads to concentric left ventricular hypertrophy

Imaging Findings

General Features
- Thickened, calcific and stenotic valve
- Systolic flow jet into the ascending aorta
- Left ventricular hypertrophy in severe AS
- Echocardiography is the most important technique for diagnosis and follow-up of patients with AS

Chest Radiography Findings
- May be normal even in severe AS
- Rounding of the left ventricular free wall
- Calcification of the valve is frequent; lack of calcification by fluoro in patient over 40 essentially eliminated the diagnosis of severe AS
- Severe calcification even in the elderly may occur in patients with mild or no AS
- Signs of left heart failure usually found in patients with concomitant mitral regurgitation

Angiography Findings
- Thickened aortic valve with systolic jet into the aorta, enlarged ascending aorta and thickened left ventricle; valvular gradient measured during catheter pull-back

Aortic Stenosis

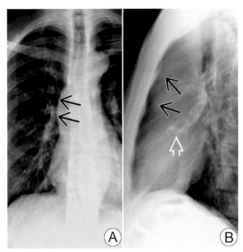

PA and lateral chest films of aortic valve stenosis. (A) Jet flow from LV through stenotic valve is responsible for dilation of ascending aorta, resulting in a bulging of the mid right mediastinal silhouette (arrows). (B) Calcification (open arrow) of the aortic valve is demonstrated, as well as the enlarged ascending aorta (arrows).

- Right and left catheterization allows valve aperture surface, cardiac function and pressure measurements and coronary arteries imaging

Echocardiography Findings
- 2D echocardiography
  - Calcified, thickened valve leaflets
  - Severity of the stenosis may be determined by the size of the orifice
  - Provides assessment of left ventricular function and mitral valve
- Doppler echocardiography
  - Systolic high velocity flow jet in the left ventricle outflow tract
  - High left ventricular-aortic pressure gradient > 50 mmHg
  - Color flow Doppler for associated MR
- Transesophageal echocardiography (TEE)
  - Decreased area of aortic valve orifice
  - Better visualization of cusps

MR Findings
- Systolic flow void (jet) into proximal aorta on cine exam
- Left ventricular hypertrophy in severe AS, enlarged when LV failure occurs

Differential Diagnosis
Degenerative Calcified Aortic Stenosis
- Marked thickening of all three leaflets
- Calcification more prominent at the base of leaflets
- Symptoms present in the 7th decade or beyond

Rheumatic Heart Disease
- Thickening predominately along the commissural edge
- Accompanies rheumatic mitral stenosis

Bicuspid Aortic Valve
- Two equal or unequal cusps
- Occurs in 2% of the population

- Symptoms present in the 4th or 5th decade
- Strong association with coarctation of the aorta

Rare Causes
- Radiation valvulitis
- Endocarditis

Pathology

General
- Thickening, fusion and calcification of aortic leaflets

Gross Pathologic, Surgical Features
- Stenotic cusps with nodular calcium depositions on the leaflets
- Calcification predominantly near the base of the valve

Microscopic Features
- Thickening and transvalvular calcification
- Inflammatory changes seen infrequently

Clinical Issues

Presentation
- Chest pain simulating coronary artery disease (CAD) occurs in > 60% of patients with severe AS
- Exertional syncope secondary to fixed cardiac output
- Symptoms of left heart failure with progressive AS
- Infectious endocarditis is a greater risk in younger patients
- Idiopathic GI bleeding can a occur in patients with calcific AS

Natural History
- Symptoms including angina, syncope and dyspnea begin in the 5th and 6th decades
- Bicuspid valve is the dominant cause below age 70
- Calcific degenerative is the dominant cause above age 70
- Survival is poor in untreated cases ranging from 2 years in patients with heart failure to 5 years in patients with angina

Treatment & Prognosis
- Surgical aortic valve replacement (AVR) is the standard treatment in patients with severe AS, associated with coronary artery bypass graft (CABG) if needed
- Mortality rate is ~ 4% for AVR; ~ 7% with accompanying CABG and ~ 10% with repair of another valve
- AVR significantly improves ventricular function and reduces clinical symptoms
- The 10 year survival rate for AVR is ~ 85%

Selected References
1. Braundwald E: Valvular Heart Disease. In: Braundwald E. Heart Disease: A Textbook of Cardiovascular Medicine 6th Ed. W.B. Saunders Company, Philadelphia, 2001
2. Rahimtolla SH: Aortic Stenosis. In: Rahimtolla SH (ed): Valvular Heart Disease and Endocarditis. Atlas of Heart Diseases. Vol. 11. Braunwald E (series editor). Current Medicine, Philadelphia, 1996

Aortic Regurgitation

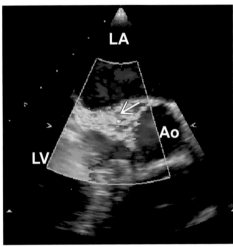

TEE showing regurgitant flow (arrow) from ascending aorta (Ao) back to left ventricle (LV) outflow tract during diastole.

Key Facts
- Secondary to diseases of the aortic valve leaflets and/or the wall of the aortic root
- Retrograde diastolic blood flow into left ventricle
- Leads to marked left ventricular enlargement

Imaging Findings
General Features
- Dilation and eccentric left ventricle (LV) hypertrophy
- Valve calcification uncommon in pure aortic regurgitation (AR)
- Dilation of aorta in aortic root disease

Chest Radiography Findings
- Minimal to massive left ventricle enlargement
- Dilation of the ascending aorta suggest aortic root disease

Echocardiography Findings
- 2D and transesophageal echocardiography (TEE)
  - Acute aortic regurgitation
    - Reduced opening motion and premature closure of valve
    - Delayed opening of mitral valve
    - Minimal dilatation of the LV cavity with normal function
  - Chronic aortic regurgitation
    - Marked dilatation of the LV cavity with decreased function
- Doppler echocardiography
  - Most sensitive method for assessment of aortic regurgitation
  - Provides estimates of regurgitant orifice size and regurgitant flow

Radionuclide Angiography Finding
- Increase in regurgitant fraction from ratio of left ventricular to right ventricular stroke volume

Left Ventricular Angiography Finding
- Regurgitant jet in LV following injection of contrast into aortic root

Aortic Regurgitation

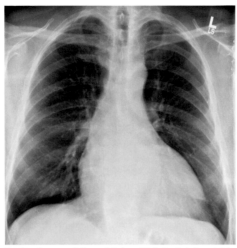

Chest plain film showing a cardiothoracic index of 0.6, due to left ventricle enlargement in a patient with aortic valve regurgitation and LV volume overload.

MR Findings
- Diastolic flow void (jet) in left ventricle
- Ventricle dilation in severe AR
- Gold standard for functional assessment; ejection fraction, LV end diastolic and end systolic volumes and LV mass

Differential Diagnosis
Aortic Root Disease
- Most common cause of pure aortic regurgitation
- Dilation of ascending aorta
- Etiologies: Degenerative, cystic medial necrosis, Marfan syndrome, dissection, osteogenesis imperfecta, aortitis

Rheumatic Heart Disease
- Thickened leaflets prevent closure during diastole
- Associated with aortic stenosis and mitral valve disease

Infective Endocarditis
- Vegetations that prevent coaptation of the cusps

Trauma
- Tear in ascending aorta
- Loss of commissural support producing prolapse of leaflet

Bicuspid Valve
- Thickening of leaflets produces incomplete closure and/or prolapse

Other Causes
- Malfunction of aortic valve replacement
- Ventricular septal defect (VSD)
- Congenital: Unicommisural, quadricuspid valves, tear in fenestrated valve

Pathology
General
- Aortic regurgitation can occur with involvement of the aortic leaflets, and ascending aorta

Aortic Regurgitation

Valve Leaflets
- Thickening, shortening and retraction of one or more leaflets
- Perforation of a valve leaflet or a vegetation that prevents coaptation of the leaflets
- Traumatic destruction of a leaflet

Ascending Aorta
- Dilatation secondary to degeneration, dissection, hypertension and infection

Myocardium
- Marked hypertrophy of the left ventricle

Clinical Issues
Presentation
- Acute aortic regurgitation
  - Signs of severe left heart failure
- Chronic aortic regurgitation
  - Progressive signs of left heart failure
  - Infectious endocarditis can exacerbate symptoms

Natural History
- Without surgery, patients with symptomatic AR live 2 to 4 years

Treatment & Prognosis
- Acute aortic regurgitation
  - Intensive medical management to stabilize for aortic valve replacement surgery
  - Five year surgical survival: 85% survival in patients with ejection fraction (EF) > 45% falling to 50% survival in patients with EF < 45%
- Chronic aortic regurgitation
  - Medical therapy: Antibiotic prophylaxis; vasodilators; calcium antagonists; arrhythmia control
  - 75% and 50% five and ten year survival
  - Surgical repair before severe left ventricular dysfunction occurs

Selected References
1. Braundwald E: Valvular Heart Disease. In Braundwald E. Heart Disease: A Textbook of Cardiovascular Medicine 6th Ed. W.B. Saunders Company, Philadelphia, 2001
2. Rahimtolla SH: Aortic Regurgitation. In Rahimtolla SH (ed): Valvular Heart Disease and Endocarditis: Atlas of Heart Diseases. Vol. 11. Braunwald E (series editor). Current Medicine, Philadelphia, 1996
3. Waller BF: Rheumatic and Nonrheumatic Conditions producing valvular heart disease. In Franfl WS and Brest AN [eds] Cardiovascular Clinics: Valvular heart disease: Comprehensive Evaluation and Management FA Davis C, Philadelphia, 1986

Mitral Stenosis

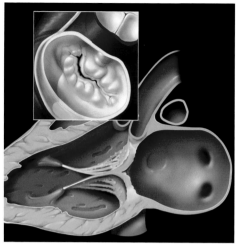

The drawing illustrates thickening of mitral valve leaflets, mitral annulus and proximal chordae tendineae, leading to mitral valve stenosis and left atrium enlargement.

Key Facts
- Rheumatic heart disease is the predominant cause
- Thickening and fusion of the mitral valve apparatus
- High velocity jet of blood ejected into left ventricle during diastole
- Frequent atrial fibrillation and associated left atrial thrombus

Imaging Findings
General Features
- Thickened, calcific and stenotic valve
- Left atrium enlargement
Chest Radiography Findings
- Left atrial enlargement on lateral or left anterior oblique (LAO) views
- Pulmonary artery, right ventricle and right atrial enlargement
- Interstitial edema with Kerley B lines
- If pulmonary hypertension, descending right pulmonary artery diameter = 16 mm
Echocardiography Findings
- 2D echocardiography
  - Increased acoustical impedance of stenotic valve
  - Fusion of leaflets with poor leaflet separation in diastole
  - Normal left ventricular function
- Doppler echocardiography
  - Diastolic high velocity flow jet in the left ventricle
  - High transvalvular pressure gradient
  - Color flow Doppler for associated valve lesions (mitral regurgitation (MR), aortic stenosis (AS) and aortic insufficiency (AI))
- Transesophageal echocardiography
  - Detailed anatomy of the mitral valve
  - Better visualization of atrial thrombus

Mitral Stenosis

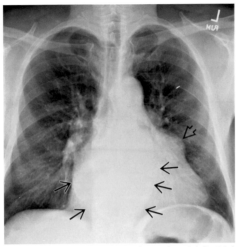

Cardiomegaly with left atrial enlargement (arrows) and left atrial appendage enlargement (open arrow). Pulmonary redistribution related to mitral valve stenosis.

Angiography Findings
- Determines the wedge pressure and indicates the degree of pulmonary hypertension, of mitral stenosis (MS) and of regurgitation
- Allows simultaneous right and left pressure measurements for direct curve comparison

MR Findings
- Diastolic flow void (jet) in left ventricle on CINE
- Left atrium enlargement

Differential Diagnosis
Rheumatic Heart Disease
- Most frequent cause of mitral stenosis > 95%
- Thickening and fusion of mitral valve apparatus

Obstruction of the Mitral Valve
- Infective endocarditis with vegetations obstructing valve orifice
- Atrial myxoma obstructing valve orifice
- Ball-valve thrombus of the left atrium

Other Causes: Rare
- Congenital mitral stenosis
- Malignant carcinoid
- Rheumatoid arthritis
- Mucopolysaccharidoses including Hunter-Hurler, Whipple's and Fabry disease

Pathology
General
- Rheumatic heart disease: Thickening, fusion and finally calcification of mitral leaflets, mitral annulus and proximal chordae tendineae

Gross Pathologic, Surgical Features
- Fusion of mitral valve apparatus

- o Commissure thickening in 30%
- o Cusps thickening in 15%
- o Chordae in 10%
- o Combination of lesions in 45%
- Valve has funnel-shaped appearance
- Thickened, adherent leaflets inhibit opening and closing of the valve
- Orifice is frequently button-hole or "fish mouth" shaped
- Calcium deposits in leaflets and occasional in annulus

Microscopic Features
- Fibrotic and calcific depositions in thickened leaflets

Clinical Issues
Presentation
- Exertional dyspnea frequently accompanied by cough and wheezing
- Hemoptysis and reduced vital capacity
- Stress-induced pulmonary edema (pregnancy)
- Progressive disease leading to right heart failure
- Chest pain simulating coronary artery disease in 15% of patients

Natural History
- Symptoms appear 15-20 years after acute rheumatic fever
- Progression more rapid in tropical and subtropical climates
- Severe disability (NYHA Class II) 5-10 after initial symptoms
- 40-60% five years survival without surgery

Treatment & Prognosis
- Medical therapy to reduce after-load and treat arrhythmias
- Percutaneous balloon mitral valvuloplasty with a mortality rate of 1-2% but relative high recurrence requiring surgery
- Surgical valvotomy with a mortality rate of 1-3% and five year survival rate > 90%
- Mitral value replacement with a mortality rate of 3-8%

Selected References
1. Braundwald E: Valvular Heart Disease. In: Braundwald E. Heart Disease: A Textbook of Cardiovascular Medicine 6th Ed. W.B. Saunders Company, Philadelphia, 2001
2. Otto CM: Mitral stenosis In: Otto CM. Valvular Heart Disease 1st Ed. W.B. Saunders Co. Philadelphia, 1999
3. Kawanishi DT et al: Mitral stenosis. In: Rahimtolla SH (ed): Valvular Heart Disease and Endocarditis. Atlas of Heart Diseases. Vol. 11. Braunwald E (series editor). Current Medicine, Philadelphia, 1996

Mitral Valve Prolapse (MVP)

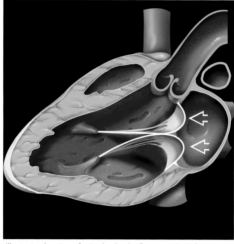

The drawing illustrates bowing of mitral valve leaflets into the left atrium (open arrows) during isovolumetric systolic left ventricle (LV) contraction.

Key Facts
- Clinical syndrome of the mitral valve producing a systolic click murmur
- Thickened, redundant mitral valve
- Systolic displacement of the valve > 2 mm above the annulus
- Moderate or severe mitral regurgitation in 10% of patients
- Most prevalent cardiac valvular abnormalities effecting 2-5% of the population: Frequency in females is 2x > males

Imaging Findings
General Features
- Thickened valve with midsystolic bowing into the left atrium
Echocardiography Findings
- 2D echocardiography
  - Thickening (3-5 mm) of one or both valve leaflets
  - Symmetrical bowing of valve leaflets > 2 mm behind the plane of the annulus
  - Asymmetrical buckling of one or both leaflets into the left atrium
  - Prolapse of the aortic and tricuspid valves in 20% of patients
- Doppler echocardiography
  - Eccentric systolic high velocity flow jet of mitral regurgitation (MR)
- Transesophageal echocardiography
  - Detailed anatomy of the mitral valve and chordae
Stress Imaging Findings
- Normal in patients with MVP and chest pain
Angiography Findings
- Buckling of mitral value
- Scalloped valve edges reflecting redundant valve tissue

Differential Diagnosis
Idiopathic
- Not associated with other diseases; most common form

Mitral Valve Prolapse (MVP)

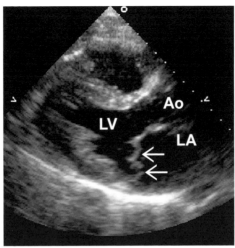

Transthoracic echocardiography showing prolapse of both mitral valve leaflets (arrows) into the left atrium (LA) during systole, Aorta (Ao).

Hereditary Connective Tissue Disease
- Marfan syndrome
- Ehlers-Danlos syndrome
- Pseudoxanthoma elasticum
- Osteogenesis imperfecta
- Von Willebrand disease
- Periarteritis nodosa

Pathology
General
- Redundant, thickening of the mitral valve
Gross Pathology
- Myxomatous proliferation of valve
Microscopic Features
- Disordered arrangement of cells
- Fragmentation of collagen network
- Endothelial disruption is frequent

Clinical Issues
Presentation
- Strong hereditary component for MVP
- 90% of Marfan syndrome and first degree relative effected
- Most patients are asymptomatic or experience syncope, palpitations and atypical chest pain
- Decreased cardiac function with severe mitral regurgitation
Natural History
- Spectrum from normal life to severe mitral regurgitation requiring surgery
- At risk for development of endocarditis, arrhythmias and spontaneous rupture of the chordae
Treatment & Prognosis
- Therapy directed toward specific symptoms

Mitral Valve Prolapse (MVP)

- Medical and surgical treatment for MVP patients with MR is the same as for patients with MR

Selected References

1. Braundwald E. Valvular Heart Disease. In: Braundwald E. Heart Disease: A Textbook of Cardiovascular Medicine 6th Ed. W.B. Saunders Company, Philadelphia, 2001
2. Becker AE et al: Pathomorphology of mitral valve prolapse. In: Boudoulas H. Woolley CF (eds): Mitral Valve: Floppy Valve, Mitral Valve Prolapse and Mitral Regurgitation. 2nd Ed., Furuta, Armonk, NY 2000
3. Boudoulas H et al: Natural History. In: Boudoulas H. Woolley CF (eds): Mitral Valve: Floppy Valve, Mitral Valve Prolapse and Mitral Regurgitation. 2nd Ed. Furuta, Armonk, NY, 2000

Mitral Regurgitation (MR)

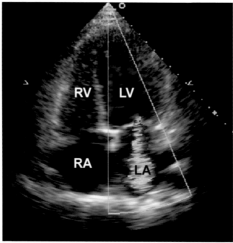

Transthoracic echocardiography apical 4-chamber view of regurgitant mitral valve. Color Doppler showing flow from left ventricle (LV) to left atrium (LA) during systole.

Key Facts
- Deformation and retraction of one or both valve cusps
- Retrograde systolic ejection of blood into left atrium
- Associated left atrium and left ventricle enlargement

Imaging Findings
General Features
- Left atrium (LA) and left ventricle (LV) enlargement
- Calcification of mitral annulus especially in elderly

Chest Radiography Findings
- Cardiomegaly with LV and LA enlargement
- Right upper lobe pulmonary vascular congestion in 10%
- Interstitial edema with Kerley B lines in acute mitral regurgitation (MR)

Echocardiography Findings
- 2D echocardiography
  - Cardiomegaly with LV and LA enlargement
  - Estimation of left ventricular function
    - Increase in LV end diastolic and end systolic volumes
    - Decrease in LV ejection fraction
- Doppler echocardiography
  - Systolic high velocity flow jet in the left atrium
  - Distance of jet correlates with the severity of regurgitation
- Transesophageal echocardiography
  - Detailed anatomy of the mitral valve especially preoperatively

Radionuclide Angiography Findings
- Increase in regurgitant fraction from ratio of left ventricular to right ventricular stroke volume

Left Ventricular Angiography Findings
- Prompt appearance of contrast in left atrium following left ventricle injection

Mitral Regurgitation (MR)

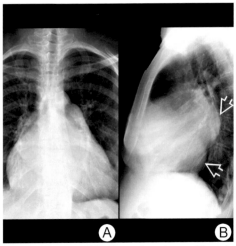

Severe cardiomegaly with enlarged left atrium and prominence of the central pulmonary vessels consistent with mitral valve regurgitation. (A) Enlargement of the pulmonary artery along the left cardiac margin on PA view. (B) Lateral view depicting LA and LV enlargement (open arrows).

MR Findings
- Systolic flow void (jet) in left atrium
- Left atrium and ventricle dilation
- Gold standard for functional assessment; ejection fraction, LV end diastolic and end systolic volumes and LV mass

Differential Diagnosis
Rheumatic Heart Disease
- Central regurgitant jet on left ventricular angiogram
- Thickened leaflets that demonstrate reduced motion
Infective Endocarditis
- Perforation of valve cusp
- Vegetations that prevents coaptation of leaflets
Collagen Vascular Disease
- Scleroderma, lupus
Cardiomyopathy
- Dilation of mitral annulus
Ischemic Heart Disease
- Papillary muscle dysfunction
Degenerative Heart Disease
- Calcific, myxomatous and Marfan syndrome

Pathology
General
- Mitral regurgitation can occur with involvement of the mitral leaflets, mitral annulus, chordae tendineae or papillary muscle
Valve Leaflets
- Rheumatic heart disease with thickening, shortening and retraction of one or more leaflets and associated shortening of the chordae tendineae

Mitral Regurgitation (MR)

- Infectious endocarditis with perforation of a valve leaflet or a vegetation that prevents coaptation of the leaflets
- Traumatic destruction of a leaflet

Mitral Annulus
- Dilation secondary to left ventricular enlargement
- Degenerative calcification in diabetes, Marfan and Hurler syndromes
  - If severe, calcific spur can project into the left ventricle

Chordae Tendineae
- Rupture secondary to rheumatic fever, endocarditis and trauma
- Posterior leaflet more frequently involved

Papillary Muscle
- Dysfunction associated with chronic ischemia and 20-30% of patients with myocardial infarction
- Involvement or infiltration with abscess, neoplasm, sarcoid, granuloma

Clinical Issues

Presentation
- Fatigue, exhaustion and right heart failure
- In chronic MR symptoms depend on the severity of the lesion, rate of progression, pulmonary artery pressure and presence of associated coronary or myocardial disease
- In acute MR, the left atrium is normal in size with an increase in pressure leading to pulmonary edema and right heart failure

Natural History
- Untreated: 40-60% mortality in 5 years

Treatment & Prognosis
- Medical therapy to reduce afterload, anticoagulation if atrial fibrillation
- Prophylaxis against endocarditis if anticipated bacteremia (dental extraction)
- Valve reconstruction or valve replacement surgery in patients with functional disability despite optimal medical management

Selected References
1.   Braundwald E: Valvular Heart Disease. In: Braundwald E. Heart Disease: A Textbook of Cardiovascular Medicine 6th ed. W.B. Saunders Company, Philadelphia, 2001
2.   Carabello B: Mitral Regurgitation. In: Rahimtolla SH (ed): Valvular Heart Disease and Endocarditis. Atlas of Heart Diseases. Vol. 11. Braunwald E (series editor). Current Medicine, Philadelphia, 1996

Pulmonary Stenosis (PS)

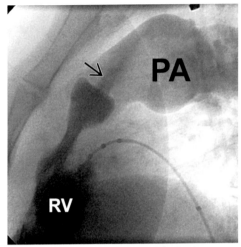

Lateral right ventricle (RV) angiogram during systole showing a cone shape jet of contrast (arrow) through the stenotic pulmonary valve, with associated ectatic pulmonary artery (PA).

Key Facts
- Congenital form is most common > 90%
- Definition: Obstructive lesion (subvalvular, valvular, supravalvular or infundibular) of the right ventricular (RV) outflow tract with post stenotic dilation
- Pressure gradient across the lesion; severe > 80 mmHg

Imaging Findings

General Features
- Thickened and stenotic valve
- Post stenotic dilation of the pulmonary artery in > 80% of patients
- Systolic flow jet into the pulmonary outflow tract
- Right ventricular hypertrophy and dysfunction in severe pulmonary stenosis (PS)

Chest Radiography Findings
- Normal heart size with dilated pulmonary artery segment in ~ 80%

Echocardiography Findings
- 2D echocardiography
  - Thickening, reduced mobility and doming of the pulmonary valve
  - Post stenotic dilation of pulmonary artery
  - Assessment of right ventricular function
- Doppler echocardiography
  - Systolic high velocity flow jet in the pulmonary outflow tract
  - High right ventricular-pulmonary artery pressure gradient

Angiography Findings
- Confirm diagnosis, measure pressures, exclude other abnormalities
- Increased trabeculation in RV

MR Findings
- Systolic flow void (jet) in pulmonary outflow tract on cine exam
- Assessment of right ventricular function

Pulmonary Stenosis (PS)

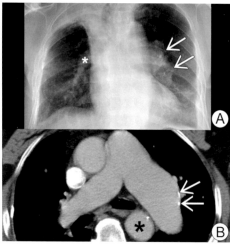

(A) The blood flow jet through the stenotic pulmonary valve is responsible for left pulmonary artery enlargement (arrows), whereas the right pulmonary artery (PA) is normal in size (*). (B) Chest CT. The left PA has nearly twice the diameter of the descending aorta (*) and demonstrates mural calcifications (arrows).

Differential Diagnosis
Congenital Heart Disease (CHD)
- Most common form of pulmonary valve disease
- 80% isolated pulmonary valve stenosis
- 20% associated with CHD including atrial septal defect (ASD), ventricular septal defect (VSD), Tetralogy of Fallot, etc.

Rheumatic Heart Disease
- Associated with mitral and aortic valve disease

Carcinoid Syndrome
- Associated with tricuspid valve disease

Pathology
General
- Various presentations

Gross Pathology
- "Dome-shaped" valve most common without calcification
- Thickened, fused leaflets, raphae extending from fused commissures
- Right ventricular hypertrophy

Microscopic Features
- Valve thickened with fibrous, myxomatous, and collagenous tissue

Clinical Issues
Presentation
- Usually asymptomatic unless severe pressure gradient (> 75 mmHg)
- Exertional dyspnea, venous congestion and right heart failure
- Cyanosis with right to left shunt

Natural History
- PS represents 7-9% of all congenital heart disease

Pulmonary Stenosis (PS)

Treatment & Prognosis
- Observation, medical management and prophylaxis in patients with gradient < 50 mmHg
- Balloon valvuloplasty or surgical valvotomy in patients with right heart failure or gradients > 50 mmHg
- Recurrence of PS ~ 15% at 10 year; hemodynamically insignificant pulmonary regurgitation in > 80% of patients post treatment

Selected References
1. Braundwald E: Valvular Heart Disease. In: Braundwald E. Heart Disease: A Textbook of Cardiovascular Medicine. 6th ed W.B. Saunders Company, Philadelphia, 2001
2. Rao PS: Pulmonary Valve Disease. In: Alpert JS, Dalen JE and Rahimtoola SH (eds): Valvular Heart Disease. 3rd ed. Lippincott William and Wilkins, Philadelphia, 2000
3. Otto CM: Right-sided Valve Disease. In: Otto CM: Valvular Heart Disease. 1st ed. W.B. Saunders Company, Philadelphia, 1999

Pulmonary Regurgitation (PR)

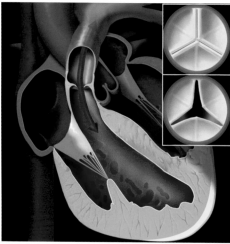

The drawing illustrates high pressure in the pulmonary artery causing diastolic pulmonary regurgitation (arrow) into the right ventricle (RV).

Key Facts
- Due to high pressure in the pulmonary artery from pulmonary arterial hypertension or secondary to mitral regurgitation or mitral stenosis
- Pulmonary artery pressure > 80 mmHg systolic unless the main pulmonary artery is markedly dilated
- Iatrogenic: Complication of balloon valvuloplasty or surgical valvotomy
- Usually benign problem

Imaging Findings
General Features
- Prominent pulmonary artery segment
- Diastolic flow jet into the right ventricle
Chest Radiography Findings
- Dilated pulmonary artery segment
- Right ventricle (RV) enlargement secondary to volume overload
Echocardiography Findings
- 2D Echocardiography
  - Dilated right ventricle in severe pulmonary regurgitation (PR)
- Doppler Echocardiography
  - Diastolic flow jet in the right ventricle
Angiography Findings
- Exclusion of other abnormalities, pressure measurements
MR Findings
- Diastolic flow void (jet) in the right ventricle on cine exam
- Assessment of right ventricular function

Differential Diagnosis
Surgical Complication
- Most common etiology

Pulmonary Regurgitation (PR)

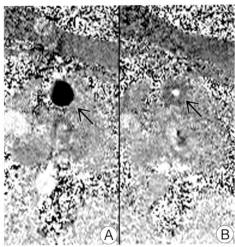

(A) Systolic and (B) Diastolic MR phase-contrast images demonstrate normal antegrade (dark) flow below the pulmonic valve during systole (black arrow, A) with a small retrograde jet (bright) of pulmonic insufficiency flow during diastole (black arrow, B).

Congenital Heart Diseases
- Absence, deformity or prolapse of the pulmonary valve

Normal Variant
- Mild PR is observed in the majority of normal subjects

Other Diseases
- Carcinoid syndrome, rheumatic, severe pulmonary hypertension

Pathology

General
- Related to surgery or primary congenital disease

Clinical Issues

Presentation
- Usually asymptomatic
- Infrequently symptoms of right ventricle volume overload

Natural History
- Rare in adults
- Generally benign course

Treatment & Prognosis
- Observation, medical management and antibiotic prophylaxis
- Surgical intervention for severe regurgitation or right heart failure

Selected References
1. Braundwald E: Valvular Heart Disease. In: Braundwald E. Heart Disease: A Textbook of Cardiovascular Medicine. 6th ed. W.B. Saunders Company, Philadelphia, 2001
2. Rao PS: Pulmonary Valve Disease In: Alpert JS, Dalen JE and Rahimtoola SH (eds): Valvular Heart Disease. 3rd ed. Lippincott William and Wilkins, Philadelphia, 2000
3. Otto CM: Right-sided Valve Disease. In: Otto CM. Valvular Heart Disease. 1st ed. W.B. Saunders Co. Philadelphia, 1999

Tricuspid Stenosis (TS)

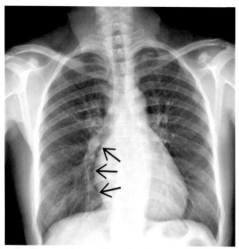

AP chest film of a 40-year-old man with combined mitral and tricuspid valve stenosis due to rheumatic heart disease. Moderate right atrium (RA) enlargement (arrows).

Key Facts
- Rheumatic heart disease is the predominant cause
- Thickening and fusion of the tricuspid valve apparatus
- Almost always accompanied with some degree of tricuspid regurgitation
- Associated with severe mitral stenosis

Imaging Findings
General Features
- Thickened and stenotic valve
- Enlarged hypertrophic right atrium
- Diastolic flow jet into the right ventricle, which remains underfilled and small
- Echocardiography finding resemble those of mitral stenosis
- Giant A waves in the jugular pulse

Chest Radiography Findings
- Marked right atrial enlargement
- Dilatation of the superior vena cava and azygos vein
- Pulmonary arteries appear normal

Angiography Findings
- Diastolic flow jet and decreased movement of valve

Echocardiography Findings
- 2D echocardiography
  - Fusion of leaflets with poor leaflet separation in diastole
  - Normal right ventricular function
- Doppler echocardiography
  - Diastolic high velocity flow jet in the right ventricle
  - High transvalvular pressure gradient
  - Most cases demonstrate associated tricuspid regurgitation
- Transesophageal echocardiography
  - Detailed anatomy of the tricuspid valve

Tricuspid Stenosis (TS)

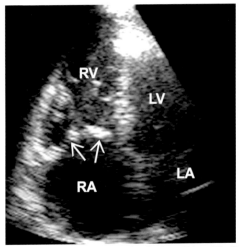

TTE apical 4-chamber view showing thickened and tethered tricuspid leaflets (arrows) in a patient with tricuspid stenosis due to carcinoid syndrome.

  o Better visualization of atrial anatomy
MR Findings
- Diastolic flow void (jet) in right ventricle
- Right atrial enlargement

Differential Diagnosis
Rheumatic Heart Disease
- Almost always the cause of tricuspid stenosis
- Thickening and fusion of tricuspid valve apparatus
- Calcification is rare
Obstruction of the Tricuspid Valve
- Right atrial tumor obstructing valve orifice
- Vegetation
- Extracardiac neoplasm
Congenital Tricuspid Stenosis
- Rare
Complication in Certain Diseases
- Carcinoid syndrome

Pathology
General
- Thickening and fusion of tricuspid leaflets
Gross Pathologic, Surgical Features
- Fusion of tricuspid valve apparatus
- Thickened, adherent leaflets inhibit opening and closing of the valve

Clinical Issues
Presentation
- Progressive fatigue and anorexia
- Hepatomegaly, ascites and peripheral edema
- Minimal pulmonary symptoms of left heart failure

Tricuspid Stenosis (TS)

Natural History
- Symptoms develop over an extended period
- Most patients have coexisting mitral valvular disease

Treatment
- Salt restriction and diuretic therapy
- Surgical repair of tricuspid stenosis is standard treatment
- Correction of other valve lesion is usually required

Selected References
1. Braundwald E: Valvular Heart Disease. In Braundwald E. Heart Disease: A Textbook of Cardiovascular Medicine. 6th Ed. W.B. Saunders Company, Philadelphia, 2001
2. Ewy GA: Tricuspid Valve Disease. In Chatterjee K, et al [ed] Cardiology: Ann Illustrated Text Reference, Vol. 2. J.B. Lippincott, Philadelphia, 1991

Tricuspid Regurgitation (TR)

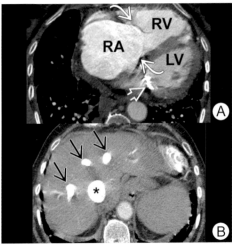

(A) Chest CT section through heart showing RA enlargement with widening of tricuspid valve annulus (curved arrows). Annular mitral valve calcifications (open arrow) are incidentally present. (B) Upper abdominal CT section showing enlarged IVC (*), hepatic veins (arrows) related to severe tricuspid valve regurgitation.

Key Facts
- Secondary to a combination of dilatation of the RV and high pressure due to severe pulmonary hypertension or RV outflow obstruction is the most common cause of tricuspid regurgitation (TR)
- Systolic pressure gradient > 55 mmHg produces functional TR
- Deformation and retraction of valve cusps in primary diseases
- Retrograde systolic ejection of blood into right atrium

Imaging Findings
General Features
- Right atrium (RA) and ventricle enlargement
- Retrograde systolic flow into the right atrium
Chest Radiography Findings
- Cardiomegaly with prominent right atrium and ventricle
- Distension of the azygous vein and superior vena cava (SVC)
Echocardiography Findings
- 2D echocardiography
  - Cardiomegaly with RA and right ventricle (RV) enlargement
  - Increase in right ventricular systolic pressure
- Doppler echocardiography
  - Systolic high velocity flow jet in the right atrium
  - Distance of jet correlates with the severity of regurgitation
Angiography Findings
- Demonstration of the TR and by measuring pressure in RV, can indicate whether the TR is primary or secondary
MR Findings
- Systolic flow void (jet) in right atrium
- Right atrium and ventricle dilation

Tricuspid Regurgitation (TR)

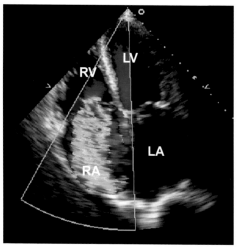

Transthoracic echo (TTE) apical 4-chamber view of tricuspid valve regurgitation. Color Doppler flow from right ventricle (RV) into right atrium (RA) during systole. Also shown: Left ventricle (LV) and left atrium (LA).

Differential Diagnosis

Primary Tricuspid Regurgitation
- Endocardial cushion defects (cleft tricuspid valve)
- Rheumatic heart disease
  - Thickening of valve leaflets and/or cordae tendineae
- Ebstein's anomaly
  - Excessive motion and delayed closure of the valve
- Carcinoid syndrome
  - Stiffened and immobile leaflets
- Infectious endocarditis
  - Vegetations on the valve leaflets (IV drug addicts)
- Trauma, atrial tumors, pacemaker leads

Secondary Tricuspid Regurgitation
- Most common cause of TR
- Right heart failure of any etiology
- Right ventricular hypertension secondary to pulmonary stenosis, primary pulmonary hypertension and mitral valve disease
- Shortly after successful mitral valvotomy for mitral stenosis in patient who had no or only slight TR preoperatively

Pathology

General
- Tricuspid regurgitation is usually secondary to diseases that cause right ventricular dilatation; it can also occur with involvement of the mitral leaflets, mitral annulus or chordae tendineae

Valve Leaflets
- Rheumatic heart disease with thickening, shortening and retraction of one or more leaflets and associate shortening of the chordae tendineae
- Infectious endocarditis with perforation of a valve leaflet or a vegetation that prevents coaptation of the leaflets

Tricuspid Regurgitation (TR)

- Traumatic destruction of a leaflet
- Carcinoid syndrome with fibrous plaques involving the leaflets

Mitral Annulus
- Dilation secondary to left ventricular enlargement

Chordae Tendineae
- Thickening and retraction due to rheumatic fever

Clinical Issues

Presentation
- TR has minimal symptoms in the absence of pulmonary hypertension
- Fatigue, exhaustion and right heart failure
- Hepatomegaly, ascites and peripheral edema

Treatment & Prognosis
- Mild TR: Medical management for patients
- Severe TR
  - Annuloplasty most common procedure; 30-40% of patients with residual TR; < 5% require valve replacement in 5 years
  - Valve replacement surgery where annuloplasty not feasible or failed; survival ~ 70% in 5 years and ~ 40% in 10 years post surgery

Selected References
1. Braundwald E: Valvular Heart Disease. In: Braundwald E. Heart Disease: A Textbook of Cardiovascular Medicine. 6th Ed. W.B. Saunders Company, Philadelphia, 2001
2. Ewy GA: Tricuspid Valve Disease. In: Alpert JS, Dalen JE and Rahimtoola SH (eds): Valvular Heart Disease. 3rd Ed. Lippincott William and Wilkins, Philadelphia, 2000
3. Otto CM: Right-sided Valve Disease. In: Otto CM. Valvular Heart Disease. 1st ed. W.B. Saunders Company, Philadelphia, 1999

Infective Endocarditis (IE)

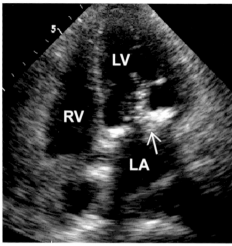

TTE apical 4-chamber view showing thickened mitral valve leaflets with vegetations (arrow) in a patient with infective endocarditis. Left ventricle (LV), right ventricle (RV), left atrium (LA).

Key Facts
- Definition: Bacterial infection of the endocardium characterized by vegetations
- Heart valves are the most common structure involved with IE
- Septic emboli and hematogenous seeding to remote sites

Imaging Findings
General Features
- Dependent on the cardiac structure involved

Echocardiography Findings
- 2D echocardiography
  - Echo dense irregular mass on the low pressure side of valve leaflet
  - Oscillation during cardiac cycle with prolapse into chamber
- Doppler echocardiography
  - Presence and severity of regurgitation and stenosis
- Transesophageal echocardiography
  - Detailed anatomy of vegetation
  - Paravalvular abscess detection

Chest Radiography Finding
- Septic pulmonary emboli especially in IV drug users

Left Ventricular Angiography Finding
- Can detect perivalvular abscess

MR Findings
- In native valves can detect myocardial abscess, aortic root aneurysm and valve dysfunction; prosthetic valves produce artifacts

Differential Diagnosis
Abnormal Valve Structure
- Thickened valve; ruptured valve or chordae, massive calcification

Pannus or Thrombus on Prosthetic Valve

Infective Endocarditis (IE)

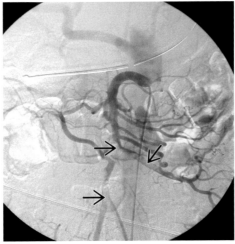

Selective superior mesenteric arteriogram in a patient with infective endocarditis, showing multiple filling defects (arrows) consistent with systemic embolization.

Pathology
General
- Amorphous mass of thrombus and inflammatory products

Gross Pathologic, Surgical Features
- Vegetation on valve leaflet or prosthetic valve
- Myocardial abscess

Microscopic Features
- Platelet and fibrin thrombus, inflammatory cells and bacteria

Clinical Issues
Presentation
- Fever, anorexia, weight loss and changing heart murmur
- Septic emboli with associated complaints, e.g., neurologic symptoms

Natural History
- 50 to 75% with prior conditions including mitral valve prolapse, rheumatic, congenital, degenerative valve disease, or prosthetic valves
- IE of prosthetic valve frequently extend to cause abscesses, fistulas and valve dehiscence resulting in paravalvular regurgitation

Treatment & Prognosis
- Long term intravenous antibiotic therapy based on microbial profile
- Surgery is recommended for failed antimicrobial therapy, lack of appropriate antibiotics (e.g., fungal), worsening congestive heart failure (CHF) due to valve dysfunction, unstable prosthesis and perivalvular invasion

Selected References
1. Karchmer AW: Infective Endocarditis. In: Braundwald E. Heart Disease: A Textbook of Cardiovascular Medicine 6th ed. W.B. Saunders Company, Philadelphia, 2001
2. Bush LM et al: Clinical Syndrome and Diagnosis. In: Kaye D (ed): Infective Endocarditis. 2nd ed. Raven Press, New York, 1992
3. Sokil AB: Cardiac imaging in infective endocarditis. In: Kaye D (ed): Infective Endocarditis. 2nd ed. Raven Press, New York, 1992

Prosthetic Valve Dysfunction

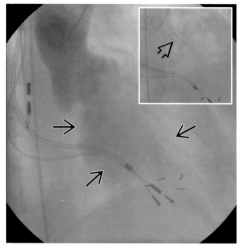

Aortic paravalvular prosthetic valve regurgitation is depicted, with contrast filling of the left ventricle (LV) (arrows). Insert showing the prosthetic valve (open arrow) during systole.

Key Facts
- Mechanical valve failure is rare: Dysfunction due to paravalvular leak thrombosis, or endocarditis
- Bioprosthetic valve failure is more common: Dysfunction due to calcification, degeneration or perforation of valve leaflet

Imaging Findings
General Features
- Dependent on type of valve

Chest Radiography Findings
- Mechanical valve: Ball or disc dislodgement
- Bioprosthetic valve: Calcification

Fluoroscopy Findings
- Mechanical valve: Rocking of a dehiscing prosthesis; strut separation

Echocardiography Findings
- 2D, Doppler and transesophageal echocardiography (TEE)
  - New findings of stenosis or regurgitation for specific valve

MR Findings
- Stenosis or regurgitation for specific valve

Angiography Findings
- Stenosis or regurgitation for specific valve

Differential Diagnosis
General Findings
- Critical to rule out other causes of heart failure from progressive stenosis and regurgitation
- Regurgitation secondary to dehiscence or disruptions of sutures

Infectious Endocarditis

Thrombosis
- ~ 20% of tricuspid valve replacement

Prosthetic Valve Dysfunction

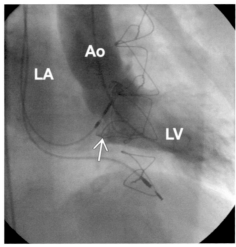

Patient with prosthetic mitral valve (arrow) replacement. During left ventricle (LV) angiogram, mitral prosthetic valve regurgitation is depicted, with complete filling of the left atrium (LA). Ascending aorta (Ao).

Other Causes of Myocardial Ischemia

Pathology
General
- Mechanical prosthesis: Disruption (rare) or paravalvular disease
- Bioprosthetic: Calcification, degeneration or perforation of valve

Clinical Issues
Presentation
- Usually gradual onset of congestive heart failure (CHF) symptoms; occasionally acute
Natural History
- Failure of mechanical valve apparatus is rare
- Overall failure of bioprosthesis is > 25% in 10 years
Treatment & Prognosis
- Medical therapy of infection, thrombosis and/or CHF
- Surgery required for non responders

Selected References
1.   Thai HM et al: Prosthetic Heart Valves. In: Alpert JS, Dalen JE and Rahimtoola SH (eds): Valvular Heart Disease. 3rd Ed. Lippincott William and Wilkins, Philadelphia, 2000
2.   Otto CM: Prosthetic Valves. In: Otto CM. Valvular Heart Disease. 1st Ed. W.B. Saunders Co. Philadelphia, 1999

Carcinoid Syndrome

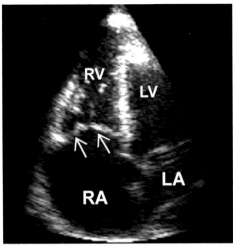

TTE apical 4-chamber view showing thickened and tethered tricuspid leaflets (arrows) in a patient with carcinoid syndrome.

Key Facts
- Rare cause of cardiac disease, yet cardiac complications are a significant cause of morbidity and mortality in this syndrome
- Secondary to hepatic metastasis from ileocecal tumors; also found in bronchial and ovarian tumors without metastasis
- Both tricuspid and pulmonary valves are involved
- Tricuspid regurgitation is the most common abnormality
- Mitral and aortic valves are spared

Imaging Findings
General Features
- Thickened leaflets similar to rheumatic involvement
- Right atrium enlargement
- Flow abnormalities related to degree of valve involvement
Chest Radiography Finding
- Right atrial enlargement
Echocardiography Finding
- 2D, Doppler and transesophageal echocardiography (TEE)
  - Tricuspid valve: Regurgitation with or without stenosis
  - Pulmonary valve: Stenosis with regurgitation less common
  - Leaflets and papillary muscles may appear highly reflective

Differential Diagnosis
Rheumatic Heart Disease
- Presence of mitral and/or aortic valve disease required
Other Causes of the Tricuspid or Pulmonary Valve Disease
- Right atrial tumor obstructing valve orifice
- Vegetation
- Extracardiac neoplasm
- Fenfluramine and phentermine usage

Carcinoid Syndrome

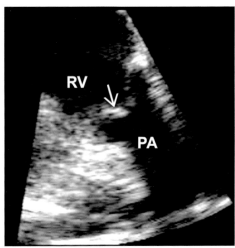

Same patient with carcinoid syndrome. Pulmonary valve sonography with thickened leaflets (arrow) and limited opening during systole consistent with related pulmonary valve stenosis.

Pathology
General
• Thickening and fusion of valve leaflets
Gross Pathologic, Surgical Features
• Coaptation of nodular thickening of valve
• Fibrous plaque coating the leaflets and papillary muscles
Microscopic Features
• Smooth muscle cells in proteoglycan matrix on valve surface

Clinical Issues
Presentation
• Syndrome: Flushing, telangiectasias, bronchospasm and diarrhea
• Progressive sign of right heart failure
Natural History
• Occurs in ~ 20% of patients with carcinoid syndrome
• Mean survival of 1 to 2 years post diagnosis
Treatment
• Medical therapy for right heart failure
• Surgical repair in severe tricuspid regurgitation

Selected References
1. Farb A et al: Pathogenesis and pathology of valvular heart disease. In: Alpert JS, Dalen JE and Rahimtoola SH (eds): Valvular Heart Disease. 3rd Ed. Lippincott William and Wilkins, Philadelphia, 2000
2. Otto CM: Right-sided valve disease. In: Otto CM. Valvular Heart Disease.1st Ed. W.B. Saunders Company, Philadelphia, 1999

Multivalvular Disease

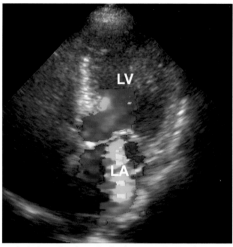

TTE Doppler apical view, showing mitral valve regurgitation during systole into the left atrium (LA).

Key Facts
- Rheumatic heart disease is the predominant cause
- Most common combination is mitral stenosis (MS) with aortic stenosis (AS) or aortic regurgitation (AR)
- Symptoms dependent on combination of valve involvement
- Marfan syndrome and connective tissue disorders can cause multivalvular regurgitation

Imaging Findings
General Features
- See findings for specific valve disease

Differential Diagnosis
Rheumatic Heart Disease
- Most frequent cause of multivalvular disease
Marfan Syndrome
- Multivalve prolapse and dilatation
Degenerative Calcification
- Frequently in mitral regurgitation (MR) and AS
Carcinoid
- Cause of combined tricuspid and pulmonic valve disease

Pathology
General
- See findings for specific valve disease

Clinical Issues
Presentation
- Depends on the severity of each of the valve lesions

Multivalvular Disease

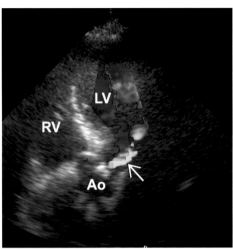

TTE Doppler apical view of the same patient during diastole, showing an aortic regurgitation (arrow).

- In situation where valve damage is equal, the proximal upstream valve determines the symptoms (tricuspid > pulmonic > mitral > aortic): The proximal valve lesion tends to mask the other lesion(s)

Natural History
- Combined aortic and mitral valve disease
  - AR and MR is the most frequent rheumatic valvular disease combination; also seen in mucopolysaccharidoses and myxomatous valve disease
  - ~ 70% of severe MS has associated mild AR
  - Severe AR and MS is uncommon
  - AS and MR can produce severe pulmonary congestion
  - The left ventricle is usually small, stiff and hypertrophic in AS and MS
- Combined tricuspid and left-sided valve disease
  - TS occurs in ~ 30% of patients with MS; women > men; may mask pulmonary symptoms
- Significant triple valve disease is rare

Treatment & Prognosis
- Double valve replacement or replacement/valvuloplasty recommended in severe cases
- Higher operative mortality
- Lower 5-year survival rates; 80% single; 60% double valve replacement

Selected References
1. Braundwald E: Valvular Heart Disease. In: Braundwald E. Heart Disease: A Textbook of Cardiovascular Medicine. 6th Ed. W.B. Saunders Company, Philadelphia, 2001
2. Paraskos JA: Combined Valve Disease. In: Alpert JS, Dalen JE and Rahimtoola SH (eds): Valvular Heart Disease. 3rd Ed. Lippincott William and Wilkins, Philadelphia, 2000

PocketRadiologist™
Cardiac
Top 100 Diagnoses

PERICARDIAL

Infectious Pericarditis

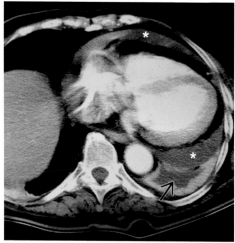

CT section showing pericardial effusion (*) in a patient with infectious pericarditis, associated with left lower lobe consolidation (arrow).

Key Facts
- Typical imaging characteristics of pericardial effusion
- Caused by bacteria, parasites, protozoa, viruses, or fungi
- Haemophilus influenza is a common cause in children

Imaging Findings
General Features
- Pericardial effusion evident by multiple imaging modalities
Chest Radiography Finding
- Flask shaped cardiac silhouette; "fat pad sign" on lateral film
Echocardiography Findings
- Effusions of varied size
- Tamponade in extreme cases
CT, MR Findings
- Typical features of pericardial effusion, tamponade, or thickened pericardium
Catheterization Findings
- Invasive data usually acquired before percutaneous or open pericardiectomy
- Features of tamponade

Differential Diagnosis
Connective Tissue Disorders
- Rheumatoid arthritis, systemic lupus, erythematosus, scleroderma
Metabolic Disorders
- Uremia
Myocardial Infarction (MI)
- 10-15% of acute MI
- Dressler's syndrome

Infectious Pericarditis

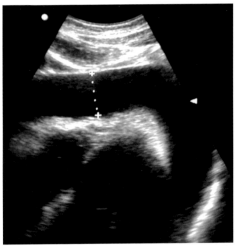

TTE showing a pericardial effusion in a patient with infectious pericarditis, as proven with subsequent pericardiocentesis.

Drugs
- Procainamide, hydralazine, isoniazid, methysergide, phenytoin, anticoagulants

Aortic Dissection
- Rupture into the pericardium

Trauma
- After pericardiotomy (5-30% of cardiac operations)

Pathology
General
- Bacterial infection is most often due to streptococci, staphylococci and gram-negative bacilli; pyogenic pericarditis is uncommon; tuberculous pericarditis (< 5%) is insidious in onset and may exist without obvious pulmonary involvement
- Acute pericarditis may be serous, fibrinous, sanguineous, hemorrhagic or purulent
- Chronic pericarditis may be serous, chylous or hemorrhagic (effusive), fibrous, adhesive or calcific (may be constrictive)

Clinical Issues
Presentation
- Pleuritic chest pain, aggravated by thoracic motion, cough and respiration
- Dyspnea, weakness, fever
- Tamponade
- ECG changes, triphasic or systolic and diastolic precordial friction rub

Natural History
- Resolve with specific antimicrobial drugs or may progress to chronic constrictive or effusive pericarditis

Treatment
- Antimicrobial drugs
- Aspirin, codeine or morphine, benzodiazepine for anxiety or insomnia

Infectious Pericarditis

- Pericardiocentesis for relief of tamponade or purulent pericarditis

Selected References
1. Spodick DH: The pericardium: A Comprehensive Textbook. Mercel Sekker, New York, 1997

Uremic Pericarditis

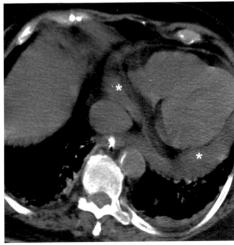

CT section demonstrating a moderate amount of low-density pericardial effusion (*), in a patient with uremia.

Key Facts
- May be a cause of hypotension in patients with renal failure, and a cause for difficult dialysis resulting from the hypotension
- An indication for more aggressive dialysis
- Typical imaging characteristics of pericardial effusion
- Can progress to tamponade
- Classical constriction is rare

Imaging Findings
General Features
- Pericardial effusion evident by multiple imaging modalities
Chest Radiography Findings
- Flask shaped cardiac silhouette; "fat pad sign" on lateral film
Echocardiography Findings
- Effusions of varied size
- Tamponade physiology in extreme cases
  - Respiratory-phasic variation
- Can be fibrinous showing fibrin strands
CT, MR Findings
- Typical features of pericardial effusion, tamponade, or thickened pericardium
Catheterization Findings
- Invasive data usually acquired before percutaneous or open pericardiectomy
- Features of tamponade

Differential Diagnosis
Other Causes of Pericarditis
- Viral, bacterial, tuberculous pericarditis
  - Especially concerning in immunocompromised state

Uremic Pericarditis

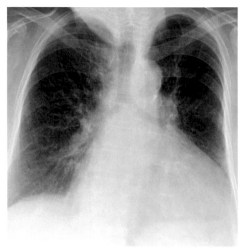

Chest film demonstrating the flask shape of the cardiac silhouette in a patient with uremia and pericardial effusion.

Aortic Dissection
- Occurs in association with poorly controlled blood pressure
- May cause hemorrhagic pericardial effusion and tamponade

Volume Overload
- Will produce transudative pericardial effusion

Myocardial Infarction
- Common in dialysis patients

Neoplastic Pericarditis
- Will not respond to dialysis

Pathology

General
- Pathogenesis uncertain
  - May be related to retained metabolites
  - Poor correlation with level of BUN or creatinine
  - In some cases may result from viral infection
  - Related to hemorrhagic diathesis
- Inflamed pericardium is usually highly vascular
- Pericardial fluid is often bloody

Clinical Issues

Presentation
- Pleuritic chest pain
- Dyspnea
- Edema, effusions
- Hypotension resulting in difficult dialysis

Natural History
- Quite variable ranging from stable mild-moderate effusion without symptoms to frank tamponade
- Constriction is uncommon, though beginning to appear with long survival on dialysis

Uremic Pericarditis

- Constriction is uncommon, though beginning to appear with long survival on dialysis
- Some effusions persist despite dialysis

Treatment
- Symptoms may be treatable with anti-inflammatory medication
- Indication for more aggressive dialysis
  - Excessive volume reduction is dangerous especially if pericardial pressure is high
- Judicious pericardiocentesis
  - Care to prevent hypotension; vasovagal or associated with cardiac dilatation

Selected References
1.   Sever MS et al: Pericarditis following Renal Transplantation. Transplantation 51:1229, 1991
2.   Spodick DH: Pericarditis in systemic disease. Cardiol Clin 8:709-16, 1990

Neoplastic Pericarditis

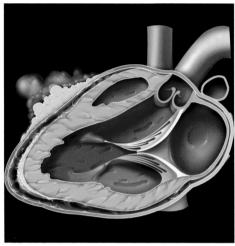

Drawing illustrating tumoral lobulated thickening of the pericardium, associated with effusion.

Key Facts
- Imaging studies will demonstrate effusion and/or mass lesions
- Varied presentation from asymptomatic to tamponade
- Effusions reaccumulate
- Cells obtained through pericardiocentesis confirm diagnosis
- Pericardial biopsy frequently necessary

Imaging Findings
General Features
- Quite varied depending on tumor type
- Mass encasing heart
- Pericardial effusion evident by multiple imaging modalities

Chest Radiography Findings
- Flask shaped cardiac silhouette in the presence of significant effusion
- Soft tissue surrounding heart

Echocardiography Findings
- Effusions of varied size
- Tamponade physiology in extreme cases
- Can demonstrate studding of pericardium with tumor
- Fibrinous adhesions of pericardium

CT, MR Findings
- Typical features of pericardial effusion, tamponade, or thickened pericardium
- Image characteristics may suggest hemopericardium
- Tumor may be visible

Catheterization Findings
- Invasive data usually acquired before percutaneous or open pericardiectomy
- Features of tamponade

Neoplastic Pericarditis

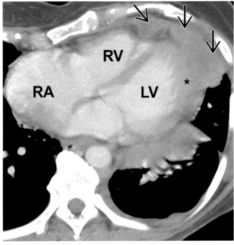

Pericardial metastasis from breast cancer. CT section showing nodular thickening of the pericardium with enhancement (arrows). Invasion of left ventricular (LV)-myocardium (*) and chest wall is suggested. The enlarged right atrium (RA) indicates component of constriction.

Differential Diagnosis
Other Causes of Pericarditis (See "Constrictive Pericarditis")

Pathology
General
- Primary tumors of the pericardium
  - Angiosarcoma and other less common sarcomas
  - Mesothelioma
  - Fibroma, lipoma
  - Pheochromocytoma, neurofibroma, neuroblastoma
  - Teratoma, thymoma
- Metastatic disease
  - Melanoma; 60% with pericardial involvement
  - Hodgkin's and non-Hodgkin's lymphoma
  - Leukemia, myeloma

Clinical Issues
Presentation
- Pleuritic chest pain
- Dyspnea, edema, effusions
- Large pericardial effusions, tamponade
- Elastic constriction resulting from tumor encasement
Natural History
- Quite variable ranging from stable mild-moderate effusion without symptoms to frank tamponade
- Poor prognosis associated with widespread metastases (~ 4 months)
  - Lymphomas frequently respond to radiation or chemotherapy
- Primary malignant tumors have poor prognosis

Neoplastic Pericarditis

Treatment
- Pericardiocentesis, with complete drainage
- Pericardiotomy (percutaneous with balloon or surgical excision) to allow drainage into the pleural space
- Treatment of primary tumor
- Extensive pericardial excision
- Pericardial peritoneal shunt, or continuous percutaneous drainage
- Sclerosing treatment in rare cases

Selected References
1. Warren WH: Malignancies involving the pericardium. Semin Thorac Cardiovas Surg 12:119-29, 2000
2. Spodick DH: Neoplastic Pericardial Disease. In: Spodick DH: The Pericardium: A Comprehensive Textbook. Marcel Dekker, New York, 301-13, 1997

Constrictive Pericarditis

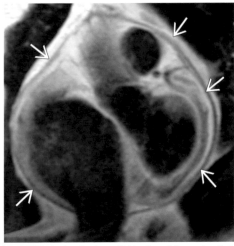

T1WI blackblood MRI, short axis view. Thickening of the pericardium (arrows) is depicted in a patient with constrictive pericarditis.

Key Facts
- Imaging demonstrates thickened pericardium
- Accentuated interventricular dependence
- Increased early diastolic filling with reduced filling beginning in mid-diastole
- Doppler flow demonstrates marked respiratory variation of filling

Imaging Findings
General Features
- Depends on level of left atrial (LA) pressure
  - Reduction in LA pressure may be necessary to reveal respiratory variation
  - Increased LA pressure reveals Kussmaul's sign and enlarged right side filling vessels

Chest Radiography Findings
- Frequently normal findings
- May show LA enlargement or Kerley B lines
  - More common with co-existent myocardial disease
- Calcification may be present
  - More common with tuberculous pericarditis, better seen on CT

Echocardiography Findings
- Paradoxical septal motion
- Abnormal inspiratory septal bounce
- Enlarged hepatic veins and venae cavae
  - Reduced diastolic collapse of venous structures

Doppler Echocardiography Findings
- Exaggerated respiratory variation of flow velocities
  - Respiratory variation of mitral velocity > 20%
  - Exaggerated variation also seen in pulmonary and hepatic veins
  - Tricuspid flow velocity increased during inspiration
  - Mitral flow velocity increased during expiration

Constrictive Pericarditis

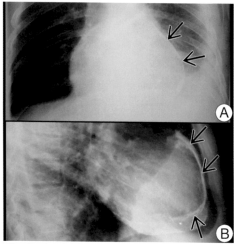

(A) PA chest film showing global cardiomegaly with discrete pericardial calcifications (arrows). Pleural effusion is present on the left side. (B) Lateral chest view with severe pericardial calcifications (arrows) in a patient with constrictive pericarditis.

- o Decreased deceleration time
- o Increased expiratory flow reversal in expiration
- False positive with severe obstructive pulmonary disease
- Respiratory variation should be demonstrated during normal relaxed respiration

MR Findings
- Pericardial thickness > 3.5 mm
  - o Early studies may have overestimated thickness by including pericardial fluid
- Chamber and septal dynamic changes on cine imaging as seen on echo

CT Findings
- Thickened pericardium
- Calcification (esp. with tuberculous pericarditis)
- Enlarged hepatic veins and venae cavae

Catheterization Findings
- Right atrial (RA) pressure: Preserved x descent and accentuated y descent
- Dip and plateau (square root sign) of left and right ventricular pressures
  - o May be masked by aggressive diuresis
- Modest elevation of right ventricular pressure (35-40 mmHg)
- Equalization of diastolic pressures (< 5 mm) of all 4 chambers
- 30% with respiratory variation of peripheral systolic pressure
- Mixed features, effusive-constrictive pericarditis
  - o Features of tamponade
  - o Demonstrates constriction after pericardiocentesis

Differential Diagnosis
Restrictive Cardiomyopathy
- Minimal variation of mitral and tricuspid flows with respiration

Constrictive Pericarditis

- Greater elevation in right ventricle (RV) pressure; > 55 mm
- Elevated pulmonary venous diastolic flow velocity without respiratory variation
- May be present in combined pericardial and myocardial disease

Obstructive Pulmonary Disease
- Marked respiratory variation of filling pressures and flows
- Response to bronchodilators will resolve hemodynamics

Cardiac Tamponade
- Frequent respiratory variation of peripheral systolic pressure
- Diastolic collapse of RA and RV

Pathology

General
- Thickened pericardium
- Fibrosis, fibrous adhesion of pericardium to the myocardium
- Leukocyte or monocyte infiltration, and vasculitis dependent on etiology
- Localized constriction may complicate diagnosis and management
- Etiology
  - Infectious
    - Viral, mycobacterial (tuberculous), fungal, bacterial
    - Rickettsial, protozoa, parasitic
    - Nocardia, actinomyces, mycoplasma, psittacosis
  - Neoplastic
  - Immunologic: Lupus, rheumatoid
  - Post-infarct
  - Post-radiation
  - Idiopathic

Clinical Issues

Presentation
- Dyspnea with exertion or at rest
- Peripheral edema
- Pleural effusion
- Ascites
- Hepatomegaly, splenomegaly
- Kussmaul's sign; increased jugular venous pressure with inspiration

Natural History
- Poor response to medical therapy
  - Diuretics, Rate control if atrial fibulations present

Treatment
- Pericardiectomy is definitive treatment
  - Need for extensive resection
- Response to treatment may not be immediate, with continued improvement over weeks to 1-2 months
- Worse prognosis with older patients, coronary disease, myocardial involvement with the disease process, or arrhythmias

Selected References
1. Myers RBH et al: Constrictive Pericarditis: Clinical and pathophysiologic characteristics. Am Heart J 138:219-32, 1999
2. Spodick DH: The pericardium: A Comprehensive Textbook. New York, Mercel Sekker, 1997

PocketRadiologist™
Cardiac
Top 100 Diagnoses

NEOPLASTIC

Atrial Myxoma

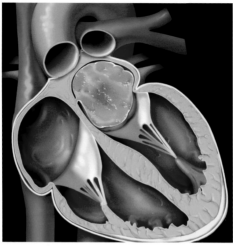

Atrial Myxoma. Note classic septal attachment of atrial myxoma. Atrial myxomas often cause secondary mitral valve obstruction.

Key Facts
- Benign intracardiac true neoplasm
- Approximately 50% of primary cardiac tumors are myxomas
- 60-80% left atrial, 20-28% in right atrium (RA), rarely in ventricles
- Typically attached to atrial septum; may prolapse through mitral valve
- 50% cause secondary mitral valve (MV) obstruction
- 50-88% are symptomatic

Imaging Findings
General Features
- Intracavitary heterogeneous mass attached to atrial septum usually at fossa ovalis

Chest Radiography Findings
- Left atrium (LA) myxoma: 50% may demonstrate signs of increased left atrial pressure, LA enlargement
  - Right retrocardiac double density, enlarged appendage, pulmonary venous hypertension (PVH)
  - Vascular redistribution or pulmonary edema
- Right atrial myxoma: 50% show calcification; enlarged inferior vena cava (IVC)/superior vena cava (SVC), azygos vein and decreased pulmonary vascularity

Echocardiography Findings
- Hyperechogenic mobile mass
- May prolapse through mitral valve (dense echoes posterior to anterior leaflet in late diastole)
- Posterior leaflet may be obscured

CT Findings
- Heterogeneous, ovoid, hypodense intraatrial lesion with lobular (75%) or smooth (25%) contour
- May be able to detect attachment site

Atrial Myxoma

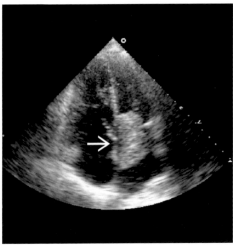

Atrial Myxoma. Four-chamber view from echocardiogram demonstrates hyperechoic mass arising from atrial septum, prolapsing into the ventricle (arrow).

- May show calcifications (RA more frequent and extensive than LA myxomas)

MR Findings
- Hypointense on T1WI
- Hyperintense on T2WI
- Positive enhancement with gadolinium

Differential Diagnosis

Thrombus
- Common, associated with atrial fibrillation and mitral valve disease
- Usually located adjacent to posterior and lateral atrial wall and appendage

Other Cardiac Tumors
- Malignant
  - Metastasis, sarcomas, lymphoma
- Benign
  - Fibroma, rhabdomyoma, lipoma, papillary fibroelastoma, etc.

Pathology

General
- 93% sporadic
- 7% familial predisposition or clinical complex, such as
  - Carney complex: Myxomas in other locations (breast, skin), spotty pigmentation (lentigines, pigmented nevi or both), endocrine overproduction (pituitary adenoma) adrenocortical disorders, testicular tumors

Gross Pathologic, Surgical Features
- 2-11 cm lobular, smooth or frond-like tumor
- Usually soft, gelatinous or friable but may be firm

Microscopic Features
- Unknown cell of origin, probably primitive mesenchymal cell

Atrial Myxoma

- Rings and nests of tumor cells and linear syncytia; variable amount of myxomatous stroma
- Hemorrhage, thrombus and hemosiderin present in 80%
- Calcification common (50%)

Clinical Issues

Presentation
- Age range 15-80 years, mean age: 50 years
- Obstructive symptoms (38%)
  - LA: Orthopnea, dyspnea
  - RA: Peripheral edema, hepatic congestion, ascites
- Constitutional (32%): Fatigue, weight loss, fever
- Other: Palpitations, arrhythmias, chest pain, embolic events

Natural History
- RA myxoma may develop septic emboli to lungs
- LA myxoma: 27% develop systemic septic emboli; 50% to brain causing mycotic aneurysms or stroke

Treatment
- Surgical resection; may need valvuloplasty

Prognosis
- Complete cure after resection in 95%
- 5% recurrence rate

Selected References
1. Grebenc ML et al: From the archives of the AFIP: Cardiac myxoma: Imaging features in 83 patients. Radiographics 22(3):673-89, 2002
2. Colucci W et al: Primary tumors of the heart. In: Braunwald E. Heart Disease: A Textbook of Cardiovascular Medicine. 6th Ed., W.B. Saunders Company, Philadelphia, 2001
3. Dähnert WF: Radiology Review Manual 4th Ed., Lippincott Williams & Wilkins, Philadelphia, 531, 1999

Cardiac Lipoma

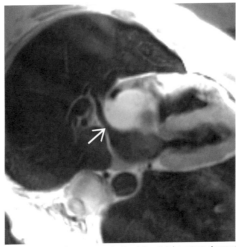

Intraatrial lipoma. T1WI shows mass in the intraatrial septum (arrow). The high signal intensity of the mass on this T1 weighted image suggests lipoma.

Key Facts
- Second most common benign primary heart tumor
- 50% subendocardial, 25% subpericardial, 25% myocardial
- Common locations are atrial septum, right atrium (RA) and left ventricle (LV)

Imaging Findings
General Features
- Fat density on CT, typical fat signal on MRI

Chest Radiography Findings
- Usually normal
- May demonstrate signs of obstruction of valve distal to lipoma if intracavitary
- May present as mass continuous with pericardium
- May have calcifications

Echocardiography Findings
- Sensitive tool to demonstrate extent and effect on cardiac function
- Echogenic sessile intraluminal mass
- TEE helpful in guiding transvenous biopsy

CT Findings
- Hypoattenuating sessile or polypoid intraluminal or epicardial mass
- Filling defect on contrast-enhanced CT

MR Findings
- Bright on T1WI
- Follows fat signal on all sequences
- Signal dropout on fat-suppressed images
- Lipomatous hypertrophy of atrial septum has bilobed appearance due to relative sparing of foramen ovale

Angiography Findings
- Intraatrial or intraventricular filling defect

Cardiac Lipoma

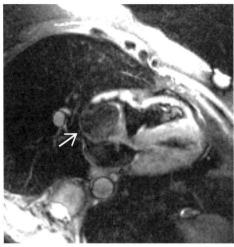

Intraatrial lipoma. Fat-suppressed T2-weighted inversion-recovery scan shows that the signal from the mass is suppressed. The exam confirms intraatrial lipoma.

Differential Diagnosis

Atrial Myxoma
- Most common benign primary tumor
- Typically left atrium
- Hypointense on T1

Other Primary Benign Tumors
- Usually readily distinguished by signal characteristics on MRI

Liposarcoma
- Very rare
- May show invasion of neighboring structures

Other Malignant Tumors
- Metastatic disease
- Usually readily distinguished by signal characteristics on MRI

Thrombus
- Most commonly in atria
- Usually does not follow signal characteristics of epicardial fat on all sequences

Pathology

General
- General path comments
  - Usually single subendocardial, myocardial or subpericardial homogeneous circumscribed tumor
- Epidemiology
  - All ages, equal sex distribution
  - More common in overweight patients

Gross Pathologic, Surgical Features
- Most are spherical, sessile or polypoid masses of homogeneous yellow fat
- Usually 1-15 cm but may be up to 2000 g

Cardiac Lipoma

Microscopic Features
- True lipomas are encapsulated and contain neoplastic mature adipocytes
- Lipomas do not contain brown fetal fat cells
- Lipomatous hypertrophy of intraatrial septum is characterized by infiltration of mature adult type or fetal fat cells between myocardial fibers with absence of capsule

Clinical Issues
Presentation
- May be asymptomatic
- May cause arrhythmias
- Subepicardial tumors may cause compression symptoms
- Intraluminal subendocardial tumors may cause location specific symptoms, such as obstruction

Treatment
- No treatment necessary if asymptomatic
- Surgical resection if symptomatic

Prognosis
- Frequently incidentally noted on autopsy
- May cause progressive obstructive or compressive symptoms requiring surgery
- Generally good outcome
- Recurrences post surgery rare

Selected References
1. Frank H: Cardiac and Paracardiac Masses. In: Manning, WJ, Pennell DJ. Cardiovascular Magnetic Resonance. Churchill Livingstone, Philadelphia, 2002
2. Colucci WS et al: Primary tumors of the heart. In: Braunwald E. Heart Disease: A Textbook of Cardiovascular Medicine. 6th ed. W.B. Saunders Company, Philadelphia, 2001
3. Grebenc ML et al: Primary cardiac and pericardial neoplasms: Radiologic-pathologic correlation. Radiographics 20(4):1073-103, 2000

Cardiac Thrombus

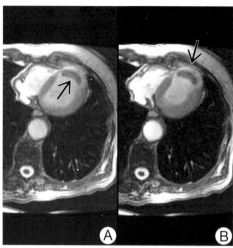

Left ventricle (LV) thrombus. (A) Diastolic FIESTA image of the left ventricular cavity in patient with apical infarct and LV thrombus (arrow). (B) Systolic image. Note the akinetic apex, with hyperenhancement due to myocardial infarction (arrow).

Key Facts
- Most frequent intracardiac mass
- Left atrium (LA) thrombus common in atrial fibrillation and mitral stenosis
- Left ventricle (LV) mural thrombus in 40-60% of patients with anterior MI if no anticoagulant therapy
- 10% of mural LV thrombi result in systemic emboli

Imaging Findings
General Features
- Intraluminal mass

Chest Radiography Finding
- May show calcifications projected over an infarcted area

Echocardiography Findings
- Preferred technique
- Ventricular thrombi usually anterior and apical
- May be laminar and adherent to wall or pedunculated and mobile echogenic masses in areas of hypokinesis
- Criteria for increased risk of embolization
  - Increased mobility, protrusion into the ventricular chamber
  - Visualization in multiple views
  - Contiguous zones of akinesis and hyperkinesis
- Experimental use of antifibrinogen labeled echogenic immunoliposomes for thrombus specific enhancement of echogenicity

CT Findings
- Higher sensitivity compared to echocardiography for detecting left atrial appendage and left lateral atrial wall thrombus

MR Findings
- Increased signal on spin-echo sequences
- Pitfall: Slow-flowing blood may also have increased signal

Cardiac Thrombus

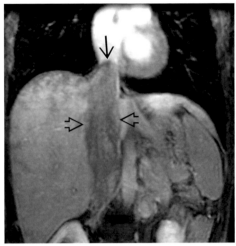

Right atrium (RA) thrombus from renal cell adenocarcinoma. Note the complete occlusion of the IVC (open arrows) with extension of the neoplastic thrombus into the right atrium at the eustachian valve (arrow). Image obtained using delayed contrast-enhanced MRA.

- Delayed contrast-enhanced spoiled gradient echo technique is highly sensitive for detecting intra-cardiac thrombus
- May be difficult to differentiate from other atrial masses
- No enhancement of thrombus with gadolinium

Angiography Findings
- Filling defect may be free floating (atrial thrombus ball)
- May be negative in case thrombus adherent to wall

Differential Diagnosis
Benign Neoplasm
- Frequently intraluminal extension
- Contrast enhancement excludes fresh thrombus

Primary or Secondary Malignancy
- Invasion of atrial or ventricular wall and contrast enhancement exclude thrombus

Pathology
Etiology
- Right atrium (RA) thrombus
  - Low cardiac output state, atrial fibrillation, central catheters or pacemaker wires, transvenous ablation procedures, embolic thrombus from deep venous thrombosis (DVT), rheumatic tricuspid stenosis, heart surgery, cardiomyopathy, extension of tumor-thrombus from kidney, liver or adrenal glands
- Right ventricle (RV) thrombus
  - Rare, same as RA thrombus
- LA thrombus
  - Atrial fibrillation most common
  - Mitral stenosis

- LV thrombus
  - Myocardial infarction (MI), LV aneurysm

<u>Gross Pathologic, Surgical Features</u>
- Freshly thrombosed blood at surface, may have organized thrombus in deep layers

<u>Microscopic Features</u>
- May be layered and adherent to myocardium
- Central layers: May be organized
  - Fibroblasts
  - Macrophages
- Superficial layers: Fibrin, platelets and red blood cells

Clinical Issues
<u>Presentation</u>
- Left chambers: Stroke, peripheral emboli
- Right chambers: Pulmonary emboli

<u>Treatment</u>
- Anticoagulation for 3-6 months with warfarin
- Aspirin may prevent further platelet deposition
- Percutaneous left atrial appendage transcatheter occlusion in high risk patients with atrial fibrillation to prevent stroke

<u>Prognosis</u>
- Mural thrombus formation within 48h to 72h post MI carries a poor prognosis from associated complications

Selected References
1. Mohiaddin RH et al: Valvular Heart Disease. In: Manning, WJ, Pennell DJ. Cardiovascular Magnetic Resonance. Churchill Livingstone, Philadelphia, 2002
2. Antman EM et al: Acute Myocardial Infarction. In: Braunwald E. Heart Disease: A Textbook of Cardiovascular Medicine. 6th ed. W.B. Saunders Company, Philadelphia, 2001
3. Dähnert WF: Radiology Review Manual 4th Ed., Lippincott Williams & Wilkins, Philadelphia, 316,1999

Cardiac Sarcoma

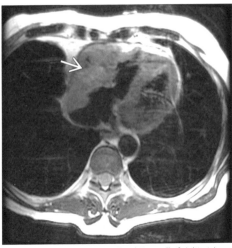

Angiosarcoma. T1WI demonstrates mass involving wall of right atrium and ventricle (arrow). Signal intensity is similar to muscle and epicenter is in myocardial wall, raising suspicion for primary cardiac malignancy. Note the broad-based origin of the lesion.

Key Facts
- Second most common primary cardiac neoplasm after myxoma
- Malignant tumor of mesenchymal cell origin
- Spectrum including angiosarcoma (37%), undifferentiated sarcomas (24%), fibrosarcoma and malignant fibrous histiocytoma (MFH) (11-24%), rhabdomyosarcoma and leiomyosarcoma, osteosarcoma
- Angiosarcoma, the most common primary malignant cardiac tumor, affects more frequently the right atrium (RA)
- MFH, osteosarcoma and leiomyosarcoma typically affect left atrium (LA)

Imaging Findings
General Features
- Invasive features characteristic

Chest Radiography Findings
- Cardiomegaly or focal cardiac mass
- Secondary findings: Congestive heart failure (CHF), pleural and pericardial effusion, atelectasis

Echocardiography Findings
- Compression and distortion of anatomy by irregular echogenic mass
- Abnormal physiology depending on tumor location and extent
- TEE useful in detection and guidance of transvenous biopsy

CT Findings
- Broad-based tumor
- Invasion of myocardium, pericardium and mediastinal structures
- May extend into great vessels
- Positive contrast enhancement, depending on vascularity
- Detection of pulmonary metastases
- Angiosarcoma typically right atrial enhancing tumors with low attenuation areas and pericardial extension

Cardiac Sarcoma

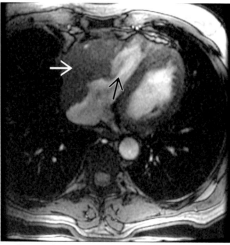

Angiosarcoma. Cine-gradient echo demonstrates mass involving wall of right atrium and ventricle (white arrow). Note flow disturbance in right ventricle (black arrow).

MR Findings
- Heterogeneous, broad-based, large masses filling most of the affected chambers
- Valvular destruction and extracardiac extension frequent
- Central tumor necrosis
- Intermediate heterogeneous signal on T1WI, higher signal on T2WI

Differential Diagnosis
Atrial Myxoma
- Most common benign primary tumor
- Typically left atrium
- Hypointense on T1W1
Other Primary Benign Tumors
- Rhabdomyoma, lipoma, hemangioma, etc.
- Usually intraluminal, no signs of invasion
Other Malignant Tumors
- Metastatic disease
- Lymphoma, pericardial mesothelioma
Thrombus
- Most commonly in atria
- No myocardial invasion

Pathology
General
- General path comments
  - Very variable appearance
  - Usually large heterogeneous invasive masses
  - May replace myocardial walls

Cardiac Sarcoma

- Etiology-Pathogenesis
  - o Unknown
- Epidemiology
  - o Mean age at presentation 41 years
  - o Extremely rare in infants and children

Gross Pathologic, Surgical Features
- Cut surfaces typically firm and heterogeneous
- May be hemorrhagic and multilobular

Microscopic Features
- Variable appearance depending on cell type
- Microscopic features parallel the corresponding soft-tissue sarcoma
- May have areas of necrosis and hemorrhage
- MFH, leiomyosarcoma and osteosarcoma may have myxoid stroma similar to that of benign myxomas

Clinical Issues

Presentation
- Usually present after 3-6 month duration of symptoms
- Dyspnea, tamponade, embolization, chest pain, arrhythmia, peripheral edema

Natural History
- Uniformly fatal

Treatment
- Aggressive surgery offers significant palliation and improves survival
- Local recurrence frequent
- Heart transplantation in rare cases

Prognosis
- Extremely poor
- Typical survival 3–12 mos; survival over 4 years has been reported
- Better prognosis if absence of metastasis, no central necrosis, low mitotic count

Selected References
1. Frank H: Cardiac and Paracardiac Masses. In: Manning, WJ, Pennell DJ. Cardiovascular Magnetic Resonance. Churchill Livingstone, Philadelphia, 2002
2. Colucci WS et al: Primary tumors of the heart. In: Braunwald E. Heart Disease: A Textbook of Cardiovascular Medicine. 6th ed. W.B. Saunders Company, Philadelphia, 2001
3. Grebenc ML et al: Primary cardiac and pericardial neoplasms: Radiologic-pathologic correlation. Radiographics 20(4):1073-103, 2000

Cardiac Metastases

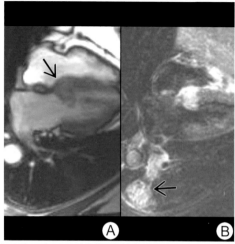

Cardiac metastatic melanoma. (A) Cine MRI demonstrates myocardial mass at base of septum (arrow). (B) Cardiac-gated T2 weighted image demonstrates increased signal at basal septum and lung mass on the bottom (arrow).

Key Facts
- 20-40 times more frequent than primary cardiac tumors
- Almost any cancer can metastasize to the heart
- Cardiac metastases are commonly found on autopsy of cancer patients
  - Leukemias (46% of autopsies), melanoma (37%), thyroid cancer (30%), lung cancer (28%), sarcomas (26%), esophageal cancer (23%), renal cell cancer (22%), lymphoma (22%), breast (21%)
- Right atrium (RA) and right ventricle (RV) much more commonly affected than left atrium (LA) and left ventricle (LV)

Imaging Findings
General Features
- Very variable imaging features, may be occult

Chest Radiography Findings
- Frequently normal
- Cardiomegaly or focal cardiac mass
- Secondary findings: Congestive heart failure (CHF), pleural and pericardial effusion, atelectasis
- Other metastases (lungs, bones)

Echocardiography Findings
- 25% no positive findings
- Pericardial effusion (50%)
- Mass or myocardial thickening evident in 40%
- May demonstrate associated thrombus

CT Findings
- Variable
- Invasion of myocardium, pericardium and mediastinal structures
- Diffuse involvement
- Positive contrast enhancement, depending on vascularity
- Secondary findings

Cardiac Metastases

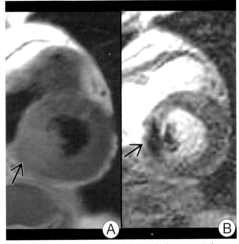

Intramyocardial metastatic melanoma. (A) T1WI shows septal myocardial mass (arrow). (B) Inversion recovery delayed-enhancement image of melanoma shows nulling of signal due to T1 shortening caused by a paramagnetic effect (arrow).

- o Pulmonary or osseous metastases
- o Pericardial effusion

MR Findings
- Similar to CT

Differential Diagnosis

Atrial Myxoma
- Most common benign primary tumor
- Typically left atrium; intraluminal
- Hypointense on T1

Other Primary Benign Tumors
- Rhabdomyoma, hemangioma etc.
- Usually intraluminal, no signs of invasion

Other Malignant Tumors
- Primary malignant cardiac tumors
  - o Lymphoma, sarcomas, pericardial mesothelioma etc.
- Direct invasion from neighboring cancers

Thrombus
- Most commonly in atria and adjacent to aneurysms
- No myocardial invasion

Pathology

General
- General path comments
  - o Very variable appearance
  - o Usually large, heterogeneous, invasive masses
  - o May replace myocardial walls
- Etiology-Pathogenesis
  - o Hematogenic spread from primary tumor
- Epidemiology

Cardiac Metastases

- o 10% incidence in cancer patients
- o Up to 40% on autopsy series

Gross Pathologic, Surgical Features
- Frequently associated sanguineous pericardial effusion
- Multiple infiltrating masses in epicardium, myocardium and endocardium

Microscopic Features
- Variable appearance depending on cell type
- Microscopic features parallel the corresponding primary tumor

Clinical Issues

Presentation
- Frequently asymptomatic
- Tamponade from hemorrhagic effusion or compressing tumor mass
- Conduction disorders
- Myocardial ischemia

Natural History
- Uniformly fatal

Treatment
- Chemotherapy for palliation
- XRT for palliation: May reduce pericardial effusion

Prognosis
- Extremely poor

Selected References
1. Meng Q et al: Echocardiographic and pathological characteristics of cardiac metastasis in patients with lymphoma. Oncology Reports 9:85-8, 2002
2. Kawamoto K etal: Antemortem diagnosis of cardiac metastasis available in a patient with Primary Toung Carcinoma. Yonago Acta Medica 44:131-6, 2001
3. Chahinian AP et al: Tumors of the heart and great vessels in Holland*Frei. Cancer Medicine. 5th Ed., BC Becker, 2000

PocketRadiologist™
Cardiac
Top 100 Diagnoses

CARDIOMYOPATHY

Hypertrophic Cardiomyopathy (HCM)

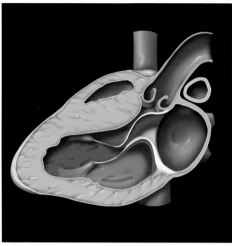

Hypertrophic cardiomyopathy with subaortic stenosis. Note thickening of anterior/ septal region of left ventricle. The thickening creates ventury effect, which causes anterior leaflet of mitral valve to displace toward septum, resulting in subaortic flow disturbance.

Key Facts
- Synonyms
  - Hypertrophic obstructive cardiomyopathy (HOCM)
  - Idiopathic hypertrophic subaortic stenosis (IHSS)
- Hallmark is myocardial hypertrophy that is inappropriate, often asymmetric, and occurs in the absence of an obvious inciting hypertrophy stimulus
- Echocardiography is diagnostic
- Leading cause of sudden cardiac death in both preadolescent and adolescent children

Imaging Findings
Chest Radiography Findings
- Variable findings, the cardiac silhouette may range from normal to markedly increased
- Left atrial enlargement frequently is observed, especially when significant mitral regurgitation is present - this is manifested by a "double-density" appearance on chest x-ray (CXR)
Two-Dimensional Echocardiography Findings
- Diagnostic for Hypertropic Cardiomyopathy (HCM); color Doppler flow studies typically reveal mitral regurgitation
- 2D images demonstrate septal thickening and systolic anterior motion (SAM) of the anterior mitral valve leaflet
- Hypertrophy does not always involve septum; lateral wall thickening is not uncommon
Radionuclide Imaging Findings
- Radionuclide imaging with thallium or technetium may show reversible defects, mostly in the absence of coronary artery disease

Hypertrophic Cardiomyopathy (HCM)

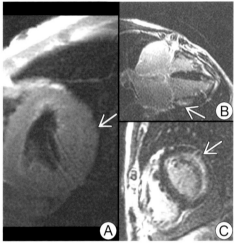

Asymmetric hypertrophic cardiomyopathy. (A) T1WI shows marked thickening of lateral wall left ventricle (arrow). (B) Long axis and (C) short axis delayed-enhancement images show myocardial fibrosis (arrows).

- These reversible defects on radionuclide scanning are more common in children and adolescents with a history of sudden death or syncope, which suggests that myocardial ischemia (MI) is a significant factor in the mechanism of the demise of younger patients with HCM

MR Findings
- Asymmetric hypertrophy
- Myocardial enhancement on delayed images
- SAM at mitral valve

Differential Diagnosis
Aortic Stenosis
- Usually supravalvular
Restrictive Cardiomyopathy
- Differentiate on echocardiography

Pathology
General
- Genetics
   o Typically is inherited in an autosomal dominant fashion with variable penetrance and variable expressivity
      ▪ Morphologic evidence of disease is found by echocardiography in approximately 25% of first-degree relatives of patients with HCM
- Etiology: The molecular basis for HCM is defects in several of the genes encoding for the sarcomeric proteins, such as myosin heavy chain, actin, tropomyosin, and titin
- The feature that has attracted the greatest attention is the dynamic pressure gradient across the left ventricle (LV) outflow tract
- HCM is reported in 0.5% of the outpatient population referred for echocardiography; the overall prevalence of HCM is low and has been estimated to occur in 0.05-0.2% of the population

Hypertrophic Cardiomyopathy (HCM)

- o Slightly more common in males than in females

<u>Microscopic Features</u>
- Myocardial hypertrophy and gross disorganization of the muscle bundles result in a characteristic whorled pattern; cell-to-cell disarray and disorganization of the myofibrillar architecture within a given cell occur in almost all patients

<u>Staging or Grading Criteria</u>
- HCM can be separated into obstructive and non-obstructive types

Clinical Issues

<u>Presentation</u>
- Death often is sudden, unexpected, and typically is associated with sports or vigorous exertion
- Symptoms can include sudden cardiac death, dyspnea, syncope and presyncope, angina, palpitations, orthopnea, paroxysmal nocturnal dyspnea, congestive heart failure, and dizziness
- Most patients are asymptomatic

<u>Treatment</u>
- Reduce ventricular contractility or increase ventricular volume, increase ventricular compliance and outflow tract dimensions, and, in the case of obstructive HCM, reduce the pressure gradient across the LV outflow tract
- Paramount to any therapy is the reduction in the risk of sudden death by identification of these patients early on and effective medical and/or surgical implantation of an automatic defibrillator

<u>Prognosis</u>
- The risk of sudden death in children is as high as 6% per year
- This is a chronic illness with life-style restrictions

Selected References
1. Braunwald E et al: Contemporary evaluation and management of hypertrophic cardiomyopathy. Circulation 106(11):1312-6, 2002
2. Wilson JM et al: Magnetic resonance imaging of myocardial fibrosis in hypertrophic cardiomyopathy. Tex Heart Inst J 29(3):176-80, 2002

Dilated Cardiomyopathy

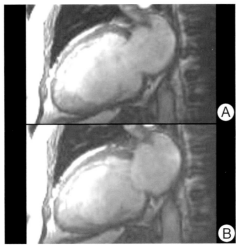

Dilated cardiomyopathy (DCM). (A) Diastolic phase and (B) systolic phase from vertical long-axis view through the left ventricle (LV) and left atrium (LA). The images demonstrate a dilated, globular configuration with global hypokinesis.

Key Facts
- Defined clinically by dilation and impaired contraction of one or both ventricles
- Common cause of congestive heart failure and is the most common diagnosis in patients referred to cardiac transplantation

Imaging Findings
Chest Radiography Finding
- Routine chest radiographs usually reveal cardiac enlargement and pulmonary redistribution suggestive of congestive heart failure on the basis of left ventricular dysfunction

Echocardiography Finding
- Patients with idiopathic DCM typically have left and right ventricular enlargement (four chamber dilatation) with decreased left ventricular function

Coronary Angiography Finding
- Patients with left ventricular dysfunction and suspected coronary artery disease should undergo coronary angiography to evaluate for areas of critical stenosis

Differential Diagnosis
Restrictive Cardiomyopathy
- Amyloid, sarcoid, hemochromatosis

Hypertrophic Cardiomyopathy
- Obstructed left ventricle (LV) outflow segment
- Familial

Pathology
General
- Genetics

Dilated Cardiomyopathy

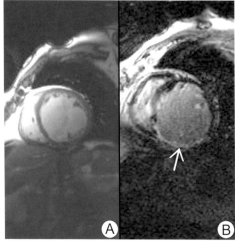

Dilated cardiomyopathy. (A) Short axis FIESTA image and (B) delayed-enhancement inversion-recovery image 10 minutes following 0.2 mmol/kg gadolinium contrast agent. The images demonstrate global thinning of the LV, with a subendocardial fibrosis involving the inferior wall (arrow).

- o Although familial aggregation of primary dilated cardiomyopathies is often unrecognized, epidemiologic studies have demonstrated that approximately 25% are inherited
- Etiology-Pathogenesis
  - o Idiopathic - 51%
  - o Idiopathic myocarditis - 9%
  - o Occult coronary disease - 8%
  - o Other identifiable causes - 32%
- Epidemiology
  - o Dilated cardiomyopathy is currently responsible for approximately 10,000 deaths and 46,000 hospitalizations each year in the United States; furthermore, idiopathic DCM is the primary indication for cardiac transplantation

Microscopic Features
- Myocyte hypertrophy and death, and replacement fibrosis with variable involvement of the conduction system

Staging or Grading Criteria
- Five phenotypes have been identified
  - o DCM with muscular dystrophy
  - o Juvenile DCM with a rapid progressive course in male relatives without muscular dystrophy
  - o DCM with segmental hypokinesis of the left ventricle
  - o DCM with conduction defects
  - o DCM with sensorineural hearing loss

Dilated Cardiomyopathy

Clinical Issues

Presentation

- Symptoms of congestive heart failure (CHF) - progressive dyspnea with exertion, impaired exercise capacity, orthopnea, paroxysmal nocturnal dyspnea, and peripheral edema - are most common

Natural History

- The dilatation often becomes severe and is invariably accompanied by hypertrophy

Treatment

- Treatment of the cause of the heart disease
- Nonpharmacologic and pharmacologic therapies directed at heart failure itself
- Consideration of systemic factors that may contribute to heart failure (e.g., anemia, infection) and of patient-related factors that might interfere with the efficacy of therapy (e.g., medical noncompliance)

Prognosis

- **NYHA functional class** — The New York Heart Association (NYHA) criteria are most often used to assess the functional class of patients with heart failure
  - Class I: No limitation during ordinary activity
  - Class II: Slight limitation by shortness of breath and/or fatigue during moderate exertion or stress
  - Class III: Symptoms with minimal exertion that interfere with normal daily activity
  - Class IV: Inability to carry out any physical activity; these patients typically have marked neurohumoral activation, muscle wasting, and reduced peak oxygen consumption

Selected References
1. Wynee J et al: The cardiomyopathies and myocarditides. In: Braunwald et al. Heart Disease: A Textbook of Cardiovascular Medicine. 6th Ed. W.B. Saunders Co. 1751-83, 2001

Restrictive Cardiomyopathy

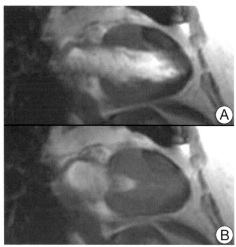

Restrictive cardiomyopathy, idiopathic. (A) Diastolic phase and (B) systolic phase of cine MRI demonstrates left ventricle (LV) hypertrophy with near-complete obliteration of the LV cavity at systole. Myocardial velocity measurements demonstrated abnormal relaxation during early diastole.

Key Facts
- Definition: Increased resistance to ventricular filling due to increased myocardial stiffness
- Classic imaging appearance
  - CXR: left atrium (LA) and left ventricle (LV) enlargement, pulmonary vascular congestion
  - Poor ventricular filling on echo or MRI
- Other key facts
  - Restrictive cardiomyopathy associated with
    - Elevated ventricular diastolic pressure
    - Increased atrial pressure
    - Global systolic function may be preserved

Imaging Findings
General Feature
- Best imaging clue: Increased left ventricular thickness and mass with infiltration of myocardium

MR Findings
- Bi-atrial enlargement
- Severe diastolic dysfunction (abnormal E/A velocity ratio, see below)
- Normal LV size
- Normal systolic function
- Specific MRI findings in "secondary" infiltrative cardiomyopathies
  - Sarcoidosis
    - T1WI + Gd: Patchy areas of high signal enhancement
    - T2WI: Patchy areas of increased signal intensity
  - Amyloidosis
    - Diffuse infiltration of myocardium on standard spin echo and functional studies
  - Hemochromatosis

Restrictive Cardiomyopathy

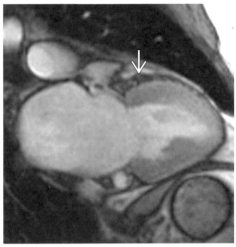

Constrictive pericarditis (CP) versus restrictive cardiomyopathy in cardiac transplant patient. Note the large left atrium due in part to the surgical anastomosis of the donor and recipient atria. Nodular pericardial thickening is present (arrow), favoring CP, which was confirmed at surgery.

- ▪ T1WI: Signal loss due to effects of iron deposition in myocardium
- ▪ T2WI: Heavy signal loss due to iron deposition in myocardium
- o Endomyocardial fibrosis
  - ▪ Primarily posterior basal or concentric wall thickening
  - ▪ Extensive subendocardial fibrosis
  - ▪ Frequent apical thrombus formation

Echocardiography Findings
- Increased left ventricular wall thickness and mass
- Normal sized left ventricular cavity
- Normal systolic function
  - o Doppler evaluation of left ventricular filling
  - o "E" (early) diastolic filling from LA to LV
  - o "A" (atrial) late diastolic filling from atrial kick
  - o E/A ratio of velocity of LV filling normally = 1.1-1.5
  - o E/A velocity ratio < 1 in early disease (impaired relaxation)
  - o "Pseudonormalization" of E/A velocity ratio with E/A > 1 in mid to late disease
  - o Advanced disease: Further reduction in ventricular compliance with E/A > 2.0

Chest Radiography Findings
- Mild cardiac enlargement
- Pulmonary venous hypertension

Differential Diagnosis
Constrictive Pericarditis
- Evidence of pericardial thickening
  - o Pericardial thickness > 4 mm on MRI
  - o Irregular appearance of pericardium, nodular thickening
  - o Pericardial calcification identified on CT

Restrictive Cardiomyopathy

- o Echocardiography findings
  - Pericardial thickening (may be difficult to detect) +/- effusion
  - Respiratory phasic variations of ventricular filling pattern

Hypertropic Cardiomyopathy
- Asymmetric pattern of hypertrophy
- Evidence of dynamic outflow subaortic obstruction
- Systolic function preserved, even late in disease

Hypertensive Heart Disease with Left Ventricular Hypertrophy
- Concentric left ventricular hypertrophy
- Mid ventricular cavity systolic obliteration
- No right ventricle (RV) involvement

Pathology
General
- General path comments
  - o Two classes of restrictive cardiomyopathy
    - Idiopathic
    - Cardiomyopathy due to infiltrative disorder
- Etiology-Pathogenesis
  - o Amyloidosis
  - o Hemochromatosis
  - o Sarcoidosis
  - o Glycogen storage diseases

Gross Pathologic, Surgical Features
- Thickening of left ventricle
- Increased left ventricular mass

Microscopic Features
- Diffuse infiltration of amyloid in amyloidosis
- Patchy infiltration of granulomas in sarcoidosis
- Extensive iron deposits in hemochromatosis
- Myocyte hypertrophy/fibrosis in endomyocardial fibrosis

Clinical Issues
Presentation
- Fatigue, weakness, anorexia, angina
- Congestive heart failure
- Physical exam demonstrates evidence of elevated central venous pressure
  - o Jugular venous distension
  - o Peripheral edema
  - o Hepatomegaly

Treatment
- Medial treatment of underlying disorder in infiltrative cardiomyopathy (CM)

Selected References
1. Friedrich MG: Cardiovascular Magnetic Resonance in Cardiomyopathies. In: Cardiovascular Magnetic Resonance, Manning WJ, Pannell DJ (ed), Churchill-Livingstone, Philadelphia. 415-8, 2002
2. Leung DY et al: Restrictive cardiomyopathy: Diagnosis and prognostic implications. In: The Practice of Clinical Echocardiography, Otto CN (ed), W.B. Saunders, Philadelphia. 473-94, 1997

Myocarditis

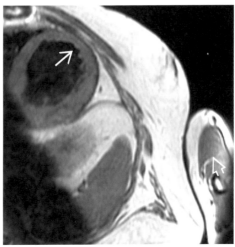

Protocol for myocarditis. Cardiac-gated T1WI of myocardium before gadolinium contrast. Myocardial enhancement is calculated by dividing the enhancement of myocardium (arrow) by the enhancement of skeletal muscle (open arrow). The normal enhancement ratio is less than 2.5.

Key Facts
- Inflammatory infiltrate of the myocardium with necrosis and/or degeneration of adjacent myocytes
- Echocardiography is performed to exclude other causes of heart failure (valvular, amyloidosis, congenital) and to evaluate the degree of cardiac dysfunction (usually diffuse hypokinesis and diastolic dysfunction)
- About 50% of the time, myocarditis is classified as "idiopathic," although a viral etiology often is suspected
  - Diagnosed by established histological, immunological, and immunochemical criteria
    - The ultimate diagnostic tool - endomyocardial biopsy - tends to be applied only to patients with major clinical manifestations such as congestive heart failure or life-threatening arrhythmias

Imaging Findings
<u>General Features</u>
- Echocardiography may allow gross localization of the extent of inflammation and distinguish between fulminant and acute myocarditis
- Antimyosin scintigraphy can identify myocardial inflammation with high sensitivity (91-100%) and negative predictive power (93-100%) but has low specificity (31-44%) and low positive predictive power (28-33%)
- Gallium scanning is used to reflect severe myocardial cellular infiltration and has a good negative predictive value, although specificity is low

<u>MR Findings</u>
- Gadolinium-enhanced MRI
  - Normal myocardial enhancement ratio < 2.5
  - Myocarditis enhancement ratio > 4.0
  - Enhancement ratio calculated by dividing the enhancement of myocardium by the enhancement of skeletal muscle.

Myocarditis

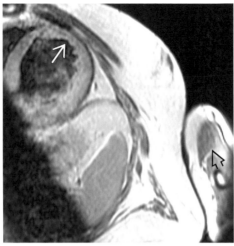

Myocarditis. Cardiac-gated T1WI of myocardium following 0.1 mmol/kg gadolinium contrast. Note the enhancement of myocardium (arrow) relative to skeletal muscle (open arrow). Patients with myocarditis show relative enhancement exceeding 4.0 (see previous figure).

Other Modality Findings
- Complete blood count - leukocytosis
- Elevated erythrocyte sedimentation rates
- Rheumatologic screening - to rule out systemic inflammatory diseases
- Elevated cardiac enzymes (creatine kinase or cardiac troponins)

Differential Diagnosis
Myocarditis
Cardiogenic Shock
- Pseudo-myocardial infarction
  - o Young patients
  - o Cardiogenic shock with classic ECG changes
  - o Febrile
  - o These patients need cardiac catheterization to rule out ischemic causes, despite the probability of myocarditis

Pathology
General
- Myocardial damage has 2 main phases
  - o Acute phase (first 2 weeks): Myocyte destruction is a direct consequence of the offending agent
  - o Chronic phase: Continuing myocyte destruction is autoimmune in nature
- Etiology-Pathogenesis
  - o Myocarditis likely is caused by a wide variety of infectious organisms, autoimmune disorders, and exogenous agents, with genetic and environmental predisposition
- Epidemiology
  - o Incidence is estimated at 1-10 per 100,000 persons

Myocarditis

Microscopic Features
- Eosin methylene blue (EMB) should reveal the simultaneous findings of lymphocyte infiltration and myocyte necrosis

Staging or Grading Criteria: WHO Marburg Classification (1996)
- Cell types: Lymphocytic, eosinophilic, neutrophilic, giant cell, granulomatous, or mixed
- Distribution: Focal (outside vessel lumen), confluent, diffuse, or reparative (in fibrotic areas)
- Amount: None (Grade 0), mild (Grade 1), moderate (Grade 2), or severe (Grade 3)

Clinical Issues

Presentation
- Acute decompensation of heart failure in a person with no other underlying cardiac dysfunction or with low cardiac risks
- Usually mild symptoms of chest pain (concurrent pericarditis), fever, sweats, chills, and dyspnea

Natural History
- Majority of cases of acute myocarditis - many of which are not detected clinically - have a benign course
- Some patients develop heart failure, serious arrhythmias, disturbances of conduction, or even circulatory collapse

Treatment
- Avoidance of exercise
- Electrocardiographic monitoring
- Antiarrhythmic drugs in selected patients
- Treatment of congestive heart failure
- Anticoagulation
- Nonsteroidal antiinflammatory drugs are not effective and may actually enhance the myocarditis and increase mortality
- Immunosuppressive therapy is not recommended for myocarditis at this time

Prognosis
- 2/3 with mild symptoms recover completely without any residual cardiac dysfunction,
- 1/3 subsequently developing dilated cardiomyopathy

Selected References
1. Friedrich MG et al: Contrast media-enhanced magnetic resonance imaging visualizes myocardial changes in the course of viral myocarditis. Circulation 97:1802-9, 1998
2. Alpert JS et al: Update in cardiology: Myocarditis. Ann Intern Med 125:40-6, 1996

Arrhythmogenic RV Dysplasia

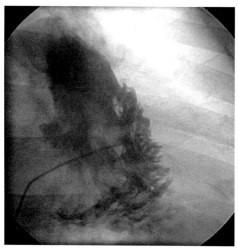

Selective right ventricular (RV) angiogram with angulated pigtail catheter. Dilated RV with thickened trabeculae and enlarged infundibulum are depicted in end diastole.

Key Facts
- Fibrofatty infiltration of the myocardium with dysfunction and occasionally associated aneurysm
- Cause of syncope, serious ventricular arrhythmias and sudden death
- Should be considered in athletes of any age as the cause of syncope or cardiovascular collapse

Imaging Findings
General Features
- Reduced right ventricular function
- Fatty infiltration of the myocardium
- Right ventricular dilatation, with wall thinning, localized aneurysms, and dyskinetic segments

Chest Radiography Findings
- Usually normal
- May show evidence of right ventricular dilatation especially on lateral view

Echocardiography Finding
- Hypokinetic and dilated right ventricle
  - Can range from mild to severe, decrease right ventricle (RV) ejection fraction

Right Ventricular Angiography Findings
- Best viewed with biplane 45 degree right and left anterior oblique
- Infundibular aneurysms
- Inferior dyskinesis
- Thickened trabeculae

CT Findings
- Dilated right ventricle
- Reduced systolic function
  - Essential to use fast techniques

Arrhythmogenic RV Dysplasia

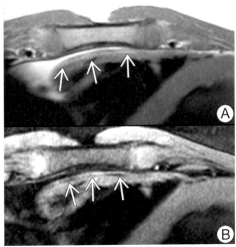

(A) T1W MRI demonstrating linear high signal (arrows) within the right ventricular free wall myocardium. (B) Fat suppressed T1W showing signal drop out of that tissue confirming presence of fat (arrows).

MR Findings
- Fatty infiltration of myocardium
- Thinned right ventricle
- Aneurysms and thickened trabeculae
- In CINE mode, altered function and dyskinesis
- No left ventricle (LV) involvement

Differential Diagnosis
Right Ventricular Infarction
- Not commonly associated with localized aneurysm formation
Volume Overloaded Right Ventricle
- Ventricular septal defect
Normal Epicardial Fat
- Thinned myocardium may make differentiation of myocardial from epicardial fat difficult
- Normal hearts may have fat intermixed with myocardial fibers

Pathology
General
- Fibrofatty infiltration of the myocardium
  - Beginning in the subepicardium and extending endocardially
  - Should have > 3% fibrous tissue and > 49% fat
  - Involves predominantly RV inflow, apex, and infundibulum
- Can involve the LV in 40-76% of autopsy cases
Familial/Genetics
- Typically autosomal dominant with incomplete penetrance
- Several genes implicated
  - Altered gene associated with plakoglobin (inadequate cell-cell adhesion)

- o Cardiac ryanodine receptor defect: Calcium released from sarcoplasmic reticulum
  - ▪ May be responsible for adrenergically mediated arrhythmias

Degenerative
- Myocyte defect due to ultrastructural abnormality
  - o Genetically determined atrophy
- Inflammation
  - o Possibly due to viral infection
- Apoptosis

Clinical Issues

Presentation
- Ventricular arrhythmias: Ventricular tachycardia with left bundle branch block (LBBB) morphology
- Syncope
- Sudden death
  - o 3-4% of sudden deaths in young athletes in the U.S.
  - o Most common cause of sudden death in young athletes in Italy
- Heart failure
  - o Isolated RV or biventricular
  - o Look for typical EKG changes of arrhyhmogenic right ventricular cardiomyopathy (ARVC) (see below)

Diagnosis
- Typical imaging findings
- EKG
  - o Epsilon waves: Small depolarization at the beginning of the ST segment
  - o T-wave inversions in early V leads
- Biopsy showing fibrofatty infiltration

Treatment & Prognosis
- Avoid vigorous athletics
- In the absence of arrhythmias, beta blocker therapy is appropriate
- Implantable cardioverter defibrillator (ICD)
  - o In patients with a history of ventricular tachyarrhythmia (VT), cardiac arrest, or syncope
  - o Antiarrhythmics may be needed for repeated discharges
    - ▪ Sotalol has shown some efficacy
    - ▪ Amiodarone not yet tested in a clinical study

Selected References
1.   Gemayel C et al: Arrhythmogenic right ventricular cardiomyopathy. J AM Coll Cardiol 38 (7): 1773-81, 2001
2.   Corrrado D et al: Arrhythmogenic right ventricular cardiomyopathy: Diagnosis, prognosis and treatment. Heart 83:588-95, 2000

PocketRadiologist™
Cardiac
Top 100 Diagnoses

CORONARY ARTERY

Anomalous Coronary Artery

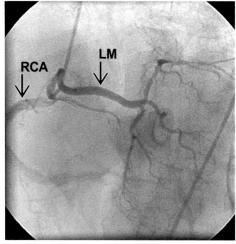

Catheterization of the right coronary artery (RCA) in LAO cranial view. Selective contrast injection showed the left main (LM) originating from the proximal RCA.

Key Facts
- Occur in 1-2% of patients
- Most often is NOT pathologic finding
- Requires diligence by angiographer to identify all branches
- For rare variants, can cause sudden death, ventricular arrhythmias, heart failure, and myocardial ischemia

Imaging Findings
General Features
- Detection and course requires multiple projections during coronary angiography
- MRI and CT have shown excellent ability for detection and characterization

Chest Radiography Finding
- Usually normal in the absence of heart failure or myocardial infarction (MI)

Echocardiography Finding
- Can occasionally detect course of proximal coronaries on transthoracic or transesophageal echocardiography

MRA Findings
- 3 dimensional or multiple 2 dimensional images may demonstrate the variants, and have the advantage of 3 dimensional and off axis display for ease of demonstration
- Can be observed with or without contrast injection

CTA Finding
- Demonstrates origin and course of anomalous artery

Differential Diagnosis
Coronary Artery Stenosis
Coronary Artery Aneurysm

Anomalous Coronary Artery

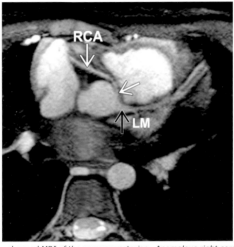

Gadolinium enhanced MRI of the coronary arteries. Anomalous right coronary artery (RCA) origin (white arrows) is depicted as it originates beside the left main (LM) (black arrow).

Pathology
<u>General</u>
- Normal histology and mechanism of sudden death not known
  - Squeezing between aorta and pulmonary artery, kinking or spasm
  - Acute angle of takeoff or slit-like origin

Clinical Issues
<u>Presentation</u>
- Incidental finding on coronary angiography
- Myocardial infarction or heart failure in an infant or young patient
- Variants are clinically significant when resulting in
  - Reduced perfusion
    - Clinical events related to ischemia resulting from constriction between the pulmonary artery (PA) and aorta, or kinking of the vessel
  - Supply of venous blood to an arterial bed
  - Production of a shunt

<u>Clinically Significant Variants</u>
- Left coronary originating from the right coronary sinus with interarterial course
- Right coronary from left sinus
- Coronary artery originating from pulmonary artery
- Coronary artery to coronary sinus shunt

<u>Treatment & Prognosis</u>
- Coronary bypass or reimplantation of coronaries above appropriate coronary sinus
- Excellent prognosis with early treatment

Anomalous Coronary Artery

Selected References
1. McConnell MV et al: Identification of anomalous coronary arteries and their anatomic course by magnetic resonance angiography. Circulation 92:3158-62, 1995
2. Taylor AJ et al: Sudden cardiac death associated with isolated congenital coronary artery anomalies. J AM Coll Cardiol 20:640-7, 1992
3. Chaitman BR et al: Angiographic, and hemodynamic findings in patients with anomalous origin of the coronary arteries. Circulation 53:122-31, 1976

Coronary Artery Aneurysm

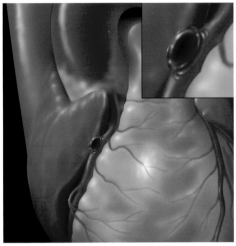

Drawing illustrates focal dilation of the proximal right coronary artery. Detailed magnification of the saccular aneurysm.

Key Facts
- Congenital or acquired
- Diagnosed on coronary angiography
- Can be detected with MR angiography or rapid CT
- Can result in thrombosis and myocardial infarction

Imaging Findings
Coronary Angiography Findings
- Fusiform and saccular dilation of proximal coronary arteries
- Sometimes associated with calcification in atherosclerosis
Echocardiography Findings
- Transthoracic and transesophageal echocardiography
  - Aneurysm detection in proximal coronaries
  - Low likelihood of detection
MR Finding
- Can detect aneurysms using coronary angiography sequence
CT Findings
- Proximal aneurysms detected using rapid CT
- Calcification frequently present with atherosclerosis etiology

Differential Diagnosis
Coronary Artery Stenosis
Anomalous Coronary Artery

Pathology
General
- Depends on etiology
- Etiology
  - Congenital
    - More common in right coronary artery (RCA)
    - May lead to thrombus formation, dissection and infarction

Coronary Artery Aneurysm

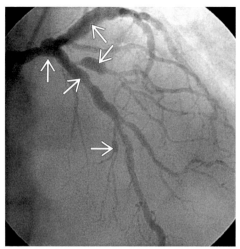

Selective left coronary artery angiogram in right anterior oblique (RAO) caudal view. Enlarged vessels with fusiform aneurysms are depicted (arrows).

- ○ Acquired
  - ▪ Atherosclerosis
  - ▪ Trauma
  - ▪ Procedural: Angioplasty, laser
  - ▪ Atherectomy
  - ▪ Arteritis
  - ▪ Mycotic emboli
  - ▪ Kawasaki's disease
  - ▪ Dissection: Primary or secondary
  - ▪ Connective tissue disease (lupus, Marfan's, Behcet's, etc.)

Clinical Issues
<u>Presentation</u>
- Myocardial infarction at young age
- Incidental finding on coronary angiography
- Myocardial ischemia as complication of exacerbation of connective tissue disease

<u>Treatment & Prognosis</u>
- For small aneurysms in the absence of evidence of ischemia, no treatment necessary
- Congenital aneurysms associated with symptoms or ischemia can be bypassed
- Covered stent graph

Selected References
1. Waller BF: Nonatherosclerotic coronary heart disease. In: Hurst JW, et al. (eds). The Heart, 9th ed. McGraw-Hill, New York, Chapter 42, 2000
2. Reidy JF et al: Transcatheter embolization in the treatment of coronary artery fistulas. J Am Coll Cardiol 18:187–192, 1991
3. Glickel SZ et al: Coronary artery aneurysm. Ann Thorac Surg 25:372–6, 1978

Coronary Calcification

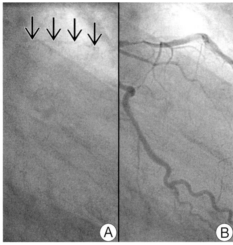

(A) Right anterior oblique (RAO) caudal selective catheterization of the left coronary artery. Native frame showing discrete calcifications along the path of the left anterior descending (LAD) (arrows). (B) Selective left main (LM) injection demonstrated a correlating proximal and mid LAD calcified stenosis.

Key Facts
- Deposition of calcium in atherosclerotic plaque
- Detected with fluoroscopy, angiography; best method is CT
- High likelihood of coronary artery dissection (CAD) and indicator of future ischemic events
- May have some use in evaluating intermediate risk
- Currently not recommended for risk stratification by the AHA, though further studies are necessary to determine potential role

Imaging Findings
General Features
- Historically has been detected with fluoroscopy
- Current methods for quantification are electron beam (EB) and helical CT
EB-CT and Helical-CT
- Bright signal > 130 HU in coronary artery segments on non contrast exam
- Current method of quantification most commonly used is Agatston method
  - o Calcium score calculated as the product of a peak attenuation factor in calcified region and area of calcium
  - o May be best technique to assess plaque burden
- Rapid simple procedure without the need for exercise or drug delivery

Differential Diagnosis
Coronary Artery Stenosis
- See "Coronary Artery Stenosis"

Pathology
General
- Calcium is a frequent finding in atherosclerotic plaque
- Represents ~ 20% of total plaque burden

144

Coronary Calcification

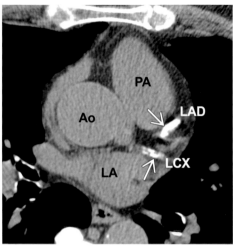

Native ECG-gated multidetector CT section at the level of the left coronary artery. Severe calcifications are demonstrated at the level of the proximal left anterior descending (LAD) and left circumflex coronary artery (LCX) (arrows).

- Represents an active osteoblastic process

Clinical Issues
- Positive studies, referred for further physician evaluation
  - Unclear which follow-up studies are appropriate
  - Need to determine pre-test probability of other examinations
- Role in medical prophylaxis unclear
- Statin therapy MAY be needed with high calcium score
- Data for normal values is age and sex dependent
- High sensitivity for detecting obstructive coronary artery disease
- Specificity in asymptomatic populations is low
- Predictive accuracy is modest (~ 70%)
- May be helpful in the emergency room setting as a predictor of CAD
- More helpful in detecting coronary artery disease than in predicting ischemic events
  - Calcium does NOT indicate the likelihood of plaque rupture
- Not necessarily helpful in diagnosing angina
  - Not adequately tested in appropriate clinical setting
  - Calcified lesions are not necessarily obstructive
  - Measures anatomy rather than physiology (flow, perfusion)
- Role vs. other risk assessments needs further study
  - One large study did NOT find incremental benefit with calcium score
  - Conflicting data exists
- Suggested as a method for following disease progression
  - Not fully tested yet

Selected References
1. O'Rourke RA et al: American College of Cardiology/American Heart Association Expert Consensus Document on Electron-Beam Computed Tomography for the Diagnosis and Prognosis of Coronary Artery Disease: Committee Members. Circulation 102:126-40, 2000
2. Budoff MJ et al: Ultrafast computed tomography as a diagnostic modality in the detection of coronary artery disease: A multicenter study. Circulation 93:898-904, 1996

Coronary Atherosclerotic Plaque

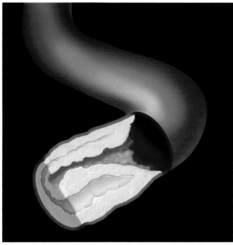

Concentric, raised, irregular lumen narrowing, which contains a lipid core.

Key Facts
- Raised irregular lumen narrowing on coronary angiography
- May not be evident on angiogram
- Can cause infarct in patients with apparently normal or minimally diseased coronary arteries
  - Plaque rupture and erosion with associated thrombus account for the bulk of acute infarcts
  - Greater than 65% of infarcts are caused in vessels with < 70% stenosis
  - Coronaries may remodel to maintain lumen size while dilating to accommodate plaque burden (Glagov effect), revealing an apparently normal coronary artery on angiography

Imaging Findings
Angiography Findings
- Concentric or eccentric lesions
- May appear normal or mild stenosis
Echocardiography Findings
- Transthoracic
  - Proximal coronary lesions occasionally detected
- Intravascular Ultrasound (IVUS)
  - Invasive technique done at the time of coronary catheterization
  - Can detect diseased segments in apparently normal coronaries
  - Normal intima not visible
  - Lesion extent: Lumen - external elastic lamina thickness
  - External elastic lamina; echo lucent border
  - Detect lesions in apparently normal vessels
    - Especially helpful in transplant vasculopathy (concentric smooth lesions)
  - Can differentiate calcific from soft plaque
  - Detect plaque rupture and erosion
  - Can guide therapy

Coronary Atherosclerotic Plaque

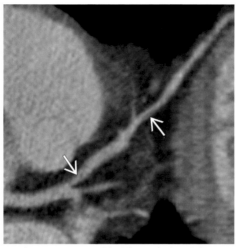

ECG-gated curved CT reconstruction of the left main (LM) and left anterior descending (LAD) coronary arteries. Some wall thickenings are demonstrated in the proximal and distal LAD, consistent with atherosclerotic plaques (arrows).

- Optimal deployment of stents; prevent incomplete apposition
- Detect dissection; guide stent deployment
- Plaque characterization still under development

MR Findings
- Allows more accurate plaque characterization
  - Spin echo T2 weighted imaging
    - Intra-plaque lipid appears bright
    - Muscularis and external elastic lamina are dark
    - Adventitial fat (triglyceride rich) is bright
  - Multispectral imaging
    - T1WI, T2WI, TOF, PDWI techniques combined to identify components
    - Identify calcium, lipid and hemorrhage
- Resolution is limited, though methods are improving
  - Intravascular MR can improve resolution and signal to noise ratio

CT Findings
- Can detect soft plaque as intermediate HU structure between adventitial fat (low HU) and contrast filled lumen (high HU)
- Unable to characterize vulnerable plaque

Angioscopy Findings
- Imaging catheter placed at the time of cardiac catheterization
- Requires saline flush to clear blood from the field
- Distinguish lesion type
  - Yellow surface: Lipid containing lesion with thin collagenous cap
  - White lesion: Thick fibrous caps, predominantly fibrous lesions
  - Yellow plaques are more likely to rupture

Optical Coherence Tomography Findings
- Examines interferogram generated by backscatter of coherent light source
- High resolution images; can measure on the scale of microns
- Requires clear field: Saline or perfluorocarbon flush

Coronary Atherosclerotic Plaque

- Penetrates 1-2 mm
- Fast imaging

Differential Diagnosis
Coronary Artery Stenosis
Coronary Artery Aneurysm

Pathology
General
- Detection of plaque
  - Multiple stages of development
    - From fatty streaks to complex lesions with hemorrhage and calcification
- Identification of vulnerable plaque
  - Thin fibrous cap
  - Large acellular lipid core
  - Inflammation in the cap and at the cap shoulders
  - Increased monocyte and macrophage content
  - Expression of matrix metalloproteinase (with collagenase activity)

Clinical Issues
Presentation
- Atherosclerotic plaque develops over several years, usually without symptoms
- Rupture or erosion of plaque accounts for the bulk of acute coronary syndromes
- Coronary arteries may appear normal on coronary angiography, yet still contain substantial plaque
Treatment & Prognosis
- Lipid lowering medication can improve lumen diameter
  - In general a minor effect
- HMG-CoA reductase inhibitors (statins) reduce coronary events in primary and secondary prevention trials
  - Several proposed plaque stabilizing properties

Selected References
1. Libby P: Current concepts of the pathogenesis of the acute coronary syndromes. Circulation 104:365-72, 2001
2. Toussaint JF et al: Magnetic resonance images lipid, fibrous, calcified, hemorrhagic, and thrombotic components of human atherosclerosis in vivo. Circulation 94:932-8, 1996
3. Falk E et al: Coronary plaque disruption. Circulation 92:657-71, 1995

Coronary Thrombosis

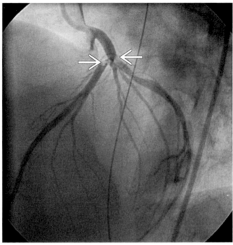

Left anterior oblique (LAO) cranial view of the left coronary artery. Thrombus is demonstrated as endoluminal filling defects (arrows) at the origin of the left anterior descending (LAD) and left circumflex (LCX) coronary arteries.

Key Facts
- Thrombus formation is the final mechanism which results in flow cessation leading to acute myocardial infarction (MI)
  - Forms the basis of thrombolytic therapy for acute MI
  - Has lead to therapies which reduce thrombogenicity for MI prevention

Imaging Findings
General Findings
- Detected at the time of x-ray contrast angiography
- Other clinical imaging modalities only detect the results of absent coronary flow, acute myocardial infarction
  - Wall motion abnormality or absent tracer extraction
  - Delayed hyperenhancement on MRI

Coronary Angiography Findings
- Smooth or round interface with contrast material
  - Occasionally contrast can seep around and outline the thrombus
- In acute setting, soft material detected upon advancement of guidewire through the material

CT, MR Imaging Findings
- Remain investigational

Differential Diagnosis
Atherosclerotic Plaque
- Most often represents the nidus for thrombus formation
  - May have rupture, erosion, or dissection leading to thrombosis
  - Sometimes important to determine relative contribution to occlusive material of thrombus vs. plaque

Embolus
- Important for secondary prevention
  - May suggest hypercoagulable state

Coronary Thrombosis

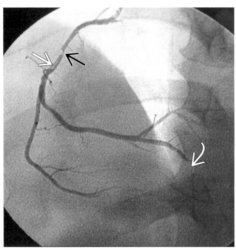

Selective left anterior oblique (LAO) cranial right coronary artery (RCA) angiogram. A severe stenosis of the RCA (black arrow) is depicted, with a poststenotic filling defect (white arrow) consistent with a thrombus. Distal thrombus embolization is shown in the proximal PDA (curved arrow) as a segmental occlusion.

Vasculitis
- May lead to artery occlusion with or without thrombus
- More often part of a systemic disease

Coronary Dissection
- Can result from percutaneous intervention
  - With advancement of the guidewire
  - During expansion of a balloon catheter

Pathology

General
- Generally white thrombus (platelet rich), with secondary areas of red thrombus formation (red cells, thrombin, fibrin)
- Various stages of thrombus maturing will affect therapy

Clinical Issues

Presentation
- Acute MI
- Sudden deterioration during percutaneous procedure

Treatment & Prognosis
- Anticoagulation to prevent further thrombus formation
- Systemic thrombolysis if catheterization lab not available
- Acute percutaneous intervention to restore flow
- Success depends on age and extent of thrombus, as well as characteristics of the underlying plaque

Selected References
1. Ramee SR et al: A randomized prospective multicenter study comparing intracoronary urokinase to rheolytic thrombectomy with the Possis Angiojet catheter for intracoronary thrombus: Final results of the Vegas-2 trial. Circulation 98:1-86, 1998
2. Kaplan BM et al: Prospective study of extraction atherectomy in patients with acute myocardial infarction. Am J Cardiol 78:383-8, 1996

Coronary Artery Stenosis

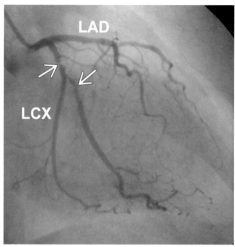

Right anterior oblique (RAO) caudal selective injection of the left coronary artery. A severe proximal left circumflex (LCX) (coronary artery) stenosis, associated with a long irregular stenosis of a large marginal branch is depicted (arrows) and responsible for a lateral left ventricle (LV) wall ischemia.

Key Facts
- Atherosclerotic plaque is the most common cause of stenosis
- Flow-limiting stenosis produces symptoms and positive stress tests
- Exercise nuclear (perfusion defect) and echocardiography (wall motion abnormality) studies can detect flow-limiting stenosis
- Coronary angiography is the gold standard to detect and quantify stenosis

Imaging Findings
General Features
- Reduced tracer uptake in perfusion dependent imaging
- Wall motion abnormalities appear during ischemia on echo and cine MRI
- Stenosis demonstrated on coronary angiogram

Chest Radiography Finding
- Usually normal in the absence of acute ischemia & congestive heart failure

Coronary Angiography Findings
- High resolution assessment of the number, location, character and severity of stenotic lesions
- Provides information of the volume of myocardium likely subtended, presence of ruptured plaque, calcification, local thrombus and collaterals

Left Ventriculography Finding
- May demonstrate region of previous infarction or stunning

Nuclear Cardiology Findings
- Thallium or technetium imaging
  - Either immediate vs. delayed thallium or immediate vs. second injection at rest technetium
  - Comparison of exercise (high-flow state) with rest (low-flow state)
  - Can use pharmacologic equivalent of exercise
    - Dobutamine and arbutamine increase cardiac work, oxygen myocardial consumption (MVO_2) and perfusion

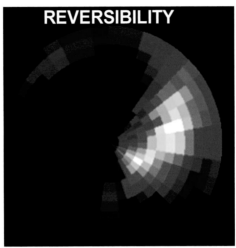

Thallium 201 scintigraphy bull's-eye substraction projection between rest and stress images confirming severe stress ischemia over the 2/3 of the lateral wall of the LV, suggesting a significant stenosis on the LCX.

- Adenosine and dipyridamole augment coronary flow and uncover lesions by demonstrating differential perfusion in normal vs. diseased territories; little change in MVO$_2$
  o Indicators of ischemic defect
    - Reduced tracer uptake, wall thinning
    - LV dilation in the stress image
    - Increased lung uptake (slow transit time)
  o Care required in interpretation
    - Apical thinning, motion artifacts and inadequate exercise

Echocardiography Findings
- Baseline study usually normal
- Stress echo most commonly performed with graded dobutamine stress
  o Increases contractility and oxygen consumption
  o Permits rapid acquisition of the stress images in several planes
  o Positive test: Angina, serious arrhythmias, new wall motion abnormality, symptoms of heart failure, significant hypotension
  o Can add atropine at max dose to increase HR to target value
  o Evaluate lack of increase in systolic function, or appearance of hypokinetic, akinetic, or dyskinetic segments

Positron Emission Tomography (PET) Findings
- PET is an excellent tool to assess perfusion, ischemia, and viability
  o Alteration in baseline and augmented perfusion: 13N-NH$_2$, 15O-H$_2$O
  o Assess metabolism: 18F-deoxyglucose, 11C-palmitate: Indicates substrate uptake and specificity
  o Marker of oxygen consumption: 11C-acetate

MR Findings
- New coronary angiography sequences available which can generate 2 or 3 dimensional images
  o Breath hold or navigator techniques with normal respiration

- o Early data suggests high sensitivity and specificity for proximal coronary lesions
- Contrast injection (Gd-DTPA) perfusion methods
  - o Can determine location, extent, and magnitude of flow limitation

CT Findings
- Presence of calcium consistent with coronary artery disease (CAD)
- CT angiograms (CTA) can detect coronary stenosis and wall lesions

Differential Diagnosis
Coronary Spasm, Syndrome X
Pericarditis, Mitral Valve Prolapse, Myocarditis, Aortic Dissection
Musculoskeletal Diseases of the Chest Wall, Shoulders, etc.
Gastrointestinal Diseases (Especially Gallbladder, Acid Reflux, Ulcer)
Cocaine Abuse

Pathology
General
- Atherosclerosis
  - o Evolution from fatty streak to raised fibrocellular plaque
  - o Components include collagenous cap, lipid core, smooth muscle cell proliferation and inflammatory cells
  - o Inflammatory cellular regions at plaque shoulders are most vulnerable to rupture

Non-Atherosclerotic Vascular Disease
- Lupus, Marfan's, Behcet's, Kawasaki's disease, aneurysm and thrombosis

Clinical Issues
Presentation
- Chest, shoulder, neck or jaw pain that is reproducible with exertion
- Dyspnea with exertion
- Screening stress-EKG examination that is positive for ischemia

Evaluation and Treatment
- Evaluation procedures are driven by pretest probability of disease and the likely need for definitive structural treatment
- Catheterization
  - o Patients who would likely require intervention (stent or surgery)
  - o Patients with persistent symptoms consistent with coronary disease
  - o Definitive diagnosis in patients with confusing noninvasive data
- Medical therapy
  - o Control of blood pressure and diabetes; smoking cessation
  - o Lower cholesterol as indicated in the ATP3 guidelines
  - o Beta blockers, nitrates and ACE inhibitors for symptoms
- Percutaneous Coronary Interventions (PCI)
  - o Angioplasty has excellent 5-year survival for single ~ 93% and multivessel disease ~ 87%
- Coronary Artery Bypass Graft (CABG) Surgery
  - o Perioperative mortality ~ 1.5-2.7% dependent on patient stability
  - o Graft patency rate at 10 years: IMA ~ 80%; saphenous vein ~ 40%

Selected References
1. Armstrong PW: Stable coronary syndromes. In Topol EJ (ed) Textbook of Cardiovascular Medicine, Lippincott-Raven, Philadelphia. 333-64, 1998
2. Beller G: Clinical Nuclear Cardiology. W.B. Saunders, Philadelphia, 1995

Ischemia RCA Stenosis

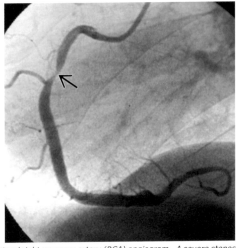

Selective lateral right coronary artery (RCA) angiogram. A severe stenosis (arrow) is demonstrated in the proximal RCA.

Key Facts
- See "Coronary Artery Stenosis"
- More difficult to diagnose because of inferior posterior location of ischemia
- Typical angina with GI symptoms more common
- Sinus and AV node ischemic symptoms more common; bradycardia

Imaging Findings
General Features
- Reduced tracer uptake in perfusion dependent imaging
- Wall motion abnormalities appear during ischemia

Chest Radiography Findings
- Usually normal in the absence of heart failure

Nuclear Cardiology Findings
- Thallium or Technetium imaging to detect reversible flow limited zones; reduced uptake, thinning
- Must differentiate inferior myocardium from diaphragm and liver; exercise reduces splanchnic flow improving contrast

Echocardiography Findings
- Reduced wall motion and wall thickening

Coronary Angiography Findings
- Stenotic lesion in the right coronary artery (RCA)
- Can evaluate collateral supply to ischemic territory

Left Ventriculography Findings
- Reduced wall motion and thickening in the infero-posterior territory

MR Findings
- Delayed first pass kinetics of contrast agent
- Contrast injection (Gd-DTPA) perfusion methods

Positron Emission Tomography (PET) Findings
- High sensitivity technique; alteration in baseline and augmented perfusion
  - 13N-Ammonia, 15O-water

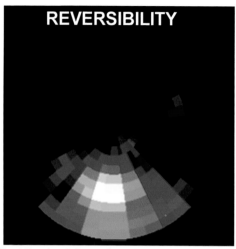

Thallium 201 scintigraphy. Bullseye substraction projection between rest and stress images demonstrating a reversible inferior stress ischemia, due to a RCA stenosis.

Differential Diagnosis
Coronary Artery Stenosis
Acute Myocardial Infarction

Pathology
Atherosclerosis
Non-Atherosclerosis Vascular Disease

Clinical Issues
Presentation
- Angina; typical chest discomfort
- Rarely, abdominal discomfort above the umbilicus
- Frequently associated with nausea or vomiting
- Can present with diaphragmatic irritation when ischemia is severe
  o Hiccups
- Bradyarrhythmias, sinus bradycardia, atrioventricular (AV) block

Evaluation and Treatment
- With mild transient symptoms, stress testing or stress imaging
- With severe persistent symptoms, may need to proceed directly to angiography

Selected References
1. Armstrong PW: Stable coronary syndromes. In: Topol EJ (ed) Textbook of Cardiovascular Medicine. Lippincott-Raven, Philadelphia. 333-64, 1998
2. Beller G: Clinical nuclear cardiology. W.B. Saunders, Philadelphia, 1995
3. Limacher MC et al: Detection of coronary artery disease with exercise two-dimensional echocardiography. Description of a clinically applicable method and comparison with radionuclide ventriculography. Circulation 67:1211-8, 1983

Left Main Coronary Stenosis

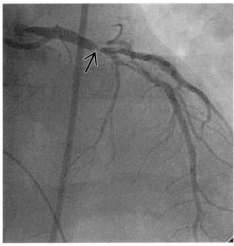

Selective left coronary artery angiogram. A severe left main (LM) stenosis (arrow) is demonstrated.

Key Facts
- Angina, characteristic symptom
- High risk lesion; minimize angiographic procedure to avoid complications
- Percutaneous treatment contraindicated; other considerations under study
- Bypass recommended over medical treatment

Imaging Findings
General Features
- Reduced tracer uptake in perfusion dependent imaging; large regional defect
- Wall motion abnormalities appear during ischemia
Chest Radiography Findings
- Usually normal in the absence of heart failure
Nuclear Cardiology Findings
- Thallium or technetium imaging to detect flow limited zones; large region of anteroapical and lateral reduced uptake, thinning
- Left ventricle (LV) dilatation may appear during stress
- Increased lung uptake with thallium imaging suggests stress-induced heart failure
Echocardiography Findings
- Reduced wall motion and wall thickening
- Chamber enlargement may be apparent
Coronary Angiography Findings
- Stenotic lesion in the left main coronary
- Ostial lesions may be difficult to locate
CT, MR Findings
- Delayed first pass kinetics of contrast agent on MR imaging
- Lesion apparent on MR and CT angiography
Positron Emission Tomography (PET) Findings
- High sensitivity for detection of ischemic territory

Left Main Coronary Stenosis

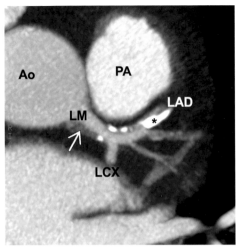

ECG-gated contrast enhanced multidetector CT MIP of the left coronary artery (LAD). The left main (LM) shows a thickened wall (arrow) responsible for a 50% stenosis. Calcifications within plaques are also demonstrated at the LM bifurcation and in the LAD (*).

Differential Diagnosis
<u>Coronary Artery Stenosis</u>
<u>Anomalous Coronary Artery</u>
<u>Coronary Artery Aneurysm</u>

Pathology
<u>Atherosclerosis</u>
<u>Non-atherosclerosis Vascular Disease</u>

Clinical Issues
<u>Presentation</u>
• Angina: Typical chest discomfort
• Heart failure: Indicative of large region of ischemia
• EKG may show ST depression and T-wave inversion of all precordial leads
<u>Evaluation</u>
• Stress test may reveal hypotension associated with heart failure symptoms
<u>Treatment</u>
• Coronary bypass surgery; best performed during the same hospitalization
• New therapies under investigation; role of stents along with new pharmacotherapy

Selected References
1. Coracciolo ES et al: Comparison of surgical and medical group survival in patients with left main equivalent coronary artery disease. Long term CASS experience. Circulation 91:2335, 1995
2. Takaro T et al: Veterans administration cooperative study of medical versus surgical treatment for stable angina-progress report. Section 3. Left main coronary artery disease. Prog Cardiovasc Dis Nov-Dec, 28(3):229-34, 1985

Coronary Artery Dissection

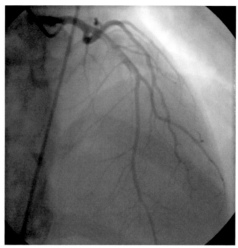

Right anterior oblique (RAO) cranial angiogram of the left coronary artery, performed after balloon angioplasty of the mid left anterior descending (LAD). Inhomogeneous filling defect of the mid LAD due to a dissection is depicted from the first to the third diagonal branches.

Key Facts
- Depict by contrast angiography and/or intravascular ultrasound (IVUS)
- May lead to acute occlusion and infarction

Imaging Findings
Coronary Angiography Findings
- Intimal flap may be apparent as linear filling defect in vessel lumen
  - May be mobile or fixed
- Linear or spiral-shaped false lumen contrast staining
- Coronary occlusion with associated filling defect

Differential Diagnosis
Thrombus
- Less often linear
- May be mobile, making flap differentiation difficult
Intraplaque Hemorrhage
- Not uncommon in complicated plaques, and as a result of plaque rupture
- May have similar clinical sequelae to dissection

Pathology
General
- Subintimal disruption
- Thrombus formation can play an intimate role in stabilizing dissection
- Etiology
  - Spontaneous dissection
  - Associated with: Postpartum state and hypertension, underlying atherosclerosis without apparent luminal narrowing, can be seen with coronary vasculitis including polyarteritis nodosa, lupus, giant cell arteritis, Kawasaki's disease and scleroderma

Coronary Artery Dissection

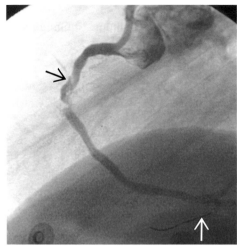

Right coronary artery (RCA) selective angiogram after ballooning of a stenosis. The guide wire (white arrow) is located in the posterior decending artery (PDA). Severe local dissection is depicted in the mid RCA. The intimal flap of the dissection (black arrow) is depicted as a lucent linear opacity within the lumen of the RCA.

Coronary Intervention
- Cannulation of vessel
- Advancing guidewire
- Balloon angioplasty
  - Can be found in ~ 60% of post-procedure examinations
  - Spiral and long (> 10 mm) dissections have worse outcomes
- Directional atherectomy followed by balloon angioplasty
- Edge dissection after stent deployment

Clinical Issues
Presentation
- Asymptomatic in most procedural complications
- Unexplained sudden heart failure in spontaneous dissection
- Acute infarction with typical presentation
  - Large dissections lead to abrupt closure in ~ 5% of cases
Treatment & Prognosis
- Many spontaneous dissections will heal spontaneously
- Thrombolytics may exacerbate dissections
- Antithrombotics and antiplatelet therapy (Gp IIb/IIIa) can reduce the risk of acute thrombosis and occlusion
- Placement of stent will tack down dissection: Definitive therapy
- Edge dissections associated with stent deployment do not require treatment

Selected References
1. Hobbs RE et al: Chronic coronary artery dissection presenting as heart failure. Circulation 100:445, 1999
2. Sanborn TA et al: The mechanism of balloon angioplasty: Evidence for formation of aneurysms in experimental atherosclerosis. Circulation 68:1136, 1983

Acute Myocardial Infarction

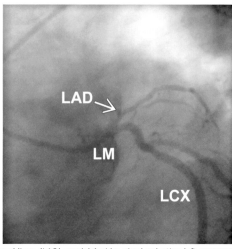

Left anterior oblique (LAO) caudal (spider view) selective left coronary angiogram. The left arterial descending (LAD) is occluded (arrow), leading to a large infarct, whereas a patent left circumflex (LCX) (coronary artery) coronary is depicted.

Key Facts
- Acute occlusion of a coronary artery
- Increased risk of ventricular arrhythmias and death
- Urgent treatment affects outcome (mortality and morbidity)
- A normal EKG does NOT exclude an acute infarct
- Imaging results are important in determining prognosis and to guide determination of culprit coronary vessel

Imaging Findings
<u>General Findings</u>
- Diminished perfusion and function to the affected area
- Reduced regional function
  - Hypokinesis: Diminished function
  - Akinesis: No function
  - Dyskinesis: Paradoxical motion
- Increased cell membrane permeability
  - Increased uptake of extracellular markers
  - Leakage of intracellular proteins
- Altered regional metabolism

<u>Chest Radiography Findings</u>
- Interstitial edema if heart failure ensues
- Abnormal cardiac silhouette
  - Changes may result form valve dysfunction
  - Size and functional deterioration may be evident on chest x-ray; left ventricle (LV) enlargement, regional aneurysm, left atrium (LA) enlargement

<u>Echocardiography Findings</u>
- 2D Echocardiography
  - Altered ventricular function
    - Decrease in ventricular ejection fraction

Acute Myocardial Infarction

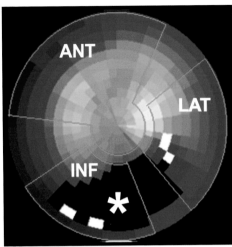

Tl 201 scintigraphy. Bullseye projection. Inferior hypoactivity is demonstrated at rest (*), consistent with an infarct. During stress no peri-infarct ischemia was demonstrated.

- - Reduced regional function; hypokinesis, akinesis, dyskinesis
  - Wall thinning
- Doppler Echocardiography
  - Mitral regurgitation (MR) with papillary muscle dysfunction

Radionuclide Angiography Findings
- Reduced overall ejection fraction
- Regional myocardial dysfunction
- Aneurysm formation; dyskinesis

Cardiac Scintigraphy Findings
- Reduced or absent tracer uptake
- Wall thinning
- Increased chamber size
- No redistribution of thallium
- No re-injection uptake of Tc99m perfusion tracer

Ventricular Angiography Findings
- Reduced regional wall motion and ejection fraction
- Reduced wall thickening, or evident thinning (dyskinesis)

Coronary Angiography Findings
- Occluded coronary artery
- Patent but tightly stenotic coronary artery, or plaque disruption
- Minimal stenosis may reflect post-infarction lysis of a large thrombus
- May show evidence of embolus

MR Findings
- Reduced wall motion and ejection fraction on cine MR
- Reduced wall thickening
- Increased signal intensity on T2 weighted imaging
- Reduced or delayed uptake of contrast agent on dynamic imaging
  - Reduced signal enhancement with T1 weighted imaging using Gd agent
- Delayed hyperenhancement
  - Central hypointense region with marked occlusion of microcirculation

o May have homogeneous hyperenhancement
- Gold standard for functional assessment; ejection fraction, LV end diastolic and end systolic volumes and LV mass

Differential Diagnosis
Old Infarction
- Wall motion abnormalities
- Persistent hyperenhancement on MRI
- Absent tracer uptake on scintigraphy
Myocarditis
- Membrane integrity is compromised
- Wall motion abnormalities
- Occasionally requires angiography for diagnosis

Pathology
General
- Myocardial necrosis
- Vascular occlusion
- Most often combined with ischemic or post-ischemic non-infarcted myocardium

Clinical Issues
Presentation
- Chest pain; substernal, pressing, occasionally radiating to the left arm
- Associated with dyspnea, nausea, palpitations, radiation to the jaw
- Any diffuse pain above the umbilicus
- Pain not sharp, or pleuritic
Treatment & Prognosis
- Medical therapy; thrombolysis in the absence of contraindications if presenting within the first 12 hours after symptoms develop
- Acute percutaneous intervention to restore flow
  o Best done within the first 3 hours
  o Optimally done with stent implantation and antiplatelet therapy with Gp IIb/IIIa inhibitor
- Acute coronary bypass is available but rarely indicated in the absence of shock and availability of percutaneous intervention
- In hospital mortality is ~ 6% while overall mortality for acute myocardial infarction (AMI) is ~ 20%

Selected References
1. Antman EM et al: Acute Myocardial Infarction In: Braundwald E. Heart Disease: A Textbook of Cardiovascular Medicine 6th ed W.B. Saunders Company, Philadelphia, 2001
2. Ryan TL et al: ACC/AHA Guidelines for the Management of Patients With Acute Myocardial Infarction. Circulation 100:1016-30, 1999
3. Topol EJ et al: Acute Myocardial Infarction. In Topol EJ. Textbook of Cardiovascular Medicine 6th ed W.B. Lippincott Raven, Philadelphia, 395-436, 1998

Infarction LAD Distribution

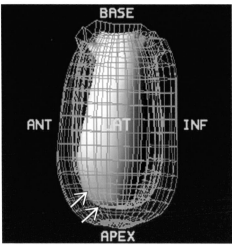

Tc 99m MIBI scintigraphy. Dynamic projection of the left ventricle (LV). In green: End diastole volume, in white: End systolic volume. A severe antero-apical hypokinesia (arrows) is demonstrated, due to infarction. Ejection fraction was calculated at 49%.

Key Facts
- Acute occlusion of the left anterior descending (LAD)
- Abnormal perfusion and function in anterior and apical regions
- Higher rate of infract expansion with potential for aneurysm and rupture
- Higher rate of left ventricle (LV) thrombus

Imaging Findings
General Findings
- Diminished perfusion, metabolism and function in anterior and apical regions

Chest Radiography Findings
- Interstitial edema if heart failure ensues
- Abnormal cardiac silhouette if anterior-apical aneurysm present

Echocardiography Findings
- 2D echocardiography
  - Altered ventricular function and anterior-apical wall thinning

Cardiac Scintigraphy Findings
- Reduced or absent tracer uptake: No redistribution of thallium
- No re-injection uptake of Tc 99m perfusion tracer

Ventricular Angiography Findings
- Reduced anterior-apical wall motion and ejection fraction
- Reduced wall thickening, or evident thinning (dyskinesis)

Coronary Angiography Findings
- Occluded LAD coronary artery
- Patent but tightly stenotic coronary artery, or plaque disruption

MR Findings
- Reduced anterior-apical perfusion and wall motion and ejection fraction on cine MR
- Increased signal intensity on T2-weighted imaging

Infarction LAD Distribution

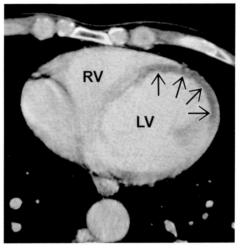

Contrast enhanced chest CT in a Marfan patient with localized supravalvular aortic dissection. The intimal flap temporarily occluded the left main (LM) inducing a left anterior descending LAD acute infarct. LV myocardial enhancement defect on the LAD territory is depicted (arrows).

- Delayed hyperenhancement

Differential Diagnosis
Coronary Artery Dissection
Old Infarction
Myocardititis

Pathology
General
- Vascular occlusion with anterior-apical necrosis
- Myocardial thinning with frequent LV thrombosis (40%)

Clinical Issues
Presentation
- Chest pain, occasionally radiating to the left arm
Treatment & Prognosis
- Thrombolysis
- Percutaneous intervention
- CABG

Selected References
1. Antman EM et al: Acute Myocardial Infarction In: Braundwald E. Heart Disease: A Textbook of Cardiovascular Medicine 6th ed. W.B. Saunders Company, Philadelphia, 2001
2. Ryan TL et al: ACC/AHA guidelines for the management of patients with acute myocardial infarction. Circulation 100:1016-30, 1999
3. Topol EJ et al: Acute Myocardial Infarction. In: Topol EJ. Textbook of Cardiovascular Medicine 6th ed W.B. Lippincott Raven, Philadelphia, 395-436, 1998

Papillary Muscle Rupture

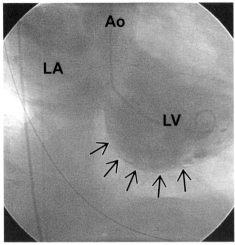

Systolic left ventricle (LV) angiogram showing severe infero-lateral hypokinesia (arrows) related to the dominant left circumflex (LCX) occlusion. Mitral valve regurgitation is observed, with contrast filling of the left atrium (LA), due to associated papillary muscle rupture.

Key Facts
- Acute hemodynamic collapse in setting of acute myocardial infarction (AMI)
- Severe mitral regurgitation: Detectable by several modalities
- Systolic murmur may be soft or absent
- Systolic function is better than anticipated, or hyperdynamic, in setting of hemodynamic compromise
- Early surgery is essential

Imaging Findings
General Features
- Severe mitral regurgitation (MR) by multiple modalities
- Reasonable systolic function

Chest Radiography Findings
- Heart failure
- Pulmonary venous congestion with signs of pulmonary edema
- Likely will **not** show evidence of left atrial enlargement

Echocardiography Findings
- Transthoracic and transesophageal echo (TEE)
  - Flail mitral leaflet
  - Papillary muscle head in left atrium (LA) or left ventricle (LV)
  - Severe mitral regurgitation on Doppler exam
    - May be low-velocity broad-based flow
  - Better than expected systolic LV function
  - TEE shows leaflets especially well, and is ideally suited for patients on ventilators or in the operating room

MR Findings
- Flow void in LA representing regurgitation
- Reasonably good LV systolic function
- Valve leaflets occasionally can be visualized in cine sequence

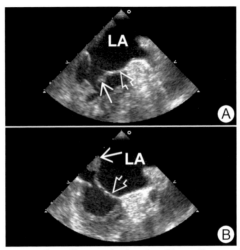

TEE showing rupture of a papillary muscle. A portion of the papillary muscle (arrows), still attached to the mitral leaflet (open arrows), is prolapsing with the flail leaflet back into the left atrium (LA). (A) Diastole, (B) systole.

Left Ventriculography Findings
- Severe MR
- Flail leaflet and papillary muscle head will frequently be apparent

Differential Diagnosis
Cardiogenic Shock with Severe Reduction in Overall Systolic Function
- Prior myocardial infarction (MI) usually present
- Multivessel or left main coronary disease
- Evident from any modality that overall function is severely reduced
Ischemic Mitral Regurgitation
- Neighboring myocardium usually shows marked wall motion abnormality
- No flail leaflet
- Lesser degree of regurgitation
Dilated Mitral Annulus
- More commonly associated with dilated LV
Chordal Rupture
- May have the same consequence as papillary muscle rupture and is difficult to distinguish
- May require TEE to distinguish from papillary muscle rupture
- Lesser degree of regurgitation is sometimes noted
Endocarditis
- Vegetation may appear as mobile structure attached to regurgitant valve
- Very different clinical setting
- Blood cultures are helpful in diagnosis

Pathology
General
- More commonly involves posterior papillary muscle, resulting from single blood supply from posterior descending coronary artery

Papillary Muscle Rupture

  o Anterior muscle is supplied by left anterior descending (LAD)
- Rupture most often at the papillary muscle head
  o May be partial or complete
- Typical necrosis apparent at site of rupture
- Infarct size may not be large

Clinical Issues
Presentation
- Recurrent chest pain
- Sudden onset heart failure
- Hemodynamic collapse
- Systolic murmur at the left lower sternal border, though may be very faint or absent
  o Absent murmur represents rapid equalization of pressure across the mitral valve
- Thrombolytics may accelerate the course of rupture
- Associations
  o Prior MI
  o Extension of MI
  o Old age
- Increased mortality

Treatment & Prognosis
- Stabilize patient with afterload reduction and diuretics
- Intraaortic balloon pump is frequently required
- Once stabilized, surgery should proceed rapidly
  o Coronary angiography may be helpful if the patient can be adequately stabilized
- Mortality rate is < 10% for mitral valve replacement
- The 10 year survival rate is 90%

Selected References
1. Lie JT et al: Sudden appearance of a systolic murmur after acute myocardial infarction. Am Heart J 90:507–12, 1975
2. Shelburne JC et al: A reappraisal of papillary muscle dysfunction: Correlative clinical and angiographic study. Am J Med 46:862–71, 1969
3. DeBusk RF et al: The clinical spectrum of papillary-muscle disease. N Engl J Med 281:1458–67, 1969

Right Ventricular Infarction

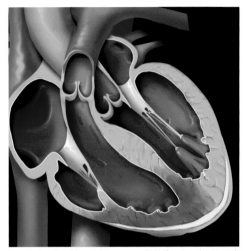

Postero-septo-apical and right ventricle myocardial infarction due to occlusion of right coronary artery (RCA) and posterior descending artery.

Key Facts
- Associated with increased mortality and morbidity
  - Ventricular arrhythmias and atrioventricle (AV) conduction abnormalities
  - Intervention is of greater importance than pure inferior infarction
- Associated with reduced cardiac output, hypotension and pump failure
- Initial diagnosis dependent on right-sided EKG leads (V3R, V4R)

Imaging Findings
General Features
- Reduced regional or global function of the right ventricle
  - Similar to effects in the left ventricle (LV)
- Reduced perfusion frequently not visible because of thin structure of the right ventricle
Chest Radiography Findings
- Hypotension in the absence of interstitial edema
- Abnormal cardiac silhouette
  - Evidence of right ventricle (RV) enlargement
Echocardiography Findings
- 2D echocardiography
  - Altered ventricular function
    - Decrease in right ventricular ejection fraction
    - Reduced regional function
- Doppler echocardiography
  - Evidence of reduced pulmonary flow
Radionuclide Angiography Findings
- Reduced RV ejection fraction
  - Regional myocardial dysfunction
Ventricular Angiography Findings
- Reduced RV regional wall motion
- Reduced RV ejection fraction

Right Ventricular Infarction

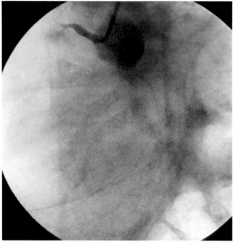

Left anterior oblique cranial right coronary artery (RCA) angiogram with a proximal thrombotic occlusion of the RCA, leading to right ventricle (RV) infarct, as well as inferior LV infarct.

Coronary Angiography Findings
- More than 90% due to RCA occlusion

Differential Diagnosis
Coronary Artery Stenosis
- See "Coronary Artery Stenosis"
Acute Valvular Regurgitation
- May NOT have a murmur
Ventricular Septal Rupture
Tamponade
- Silent cardiac exam; elevated jugular venous pressure

Pathology
General
- Myocardial necrosis
- Coronary occlusion

Clinical Issues
Presentation
- Chest pain, hypotension and ventricular arrhythmias
- EKG shows ST elevation in the right ventricular leads (V3R, V4R)
Treatment & Prognosis
- Volume expansion is critical to medical treatment
- Acute reperfusion; percutaneous intervention or thrombolysis

Selected References
1.   Mehta SR et al: Impact of right ventricular involvement on mortality and morbidity in patients with inferior myocardial infarction. J Am Coll Cardiology 37:37-43, 2001
2.   Jugdutt BI: Right ventricular infarction: Contribution of echocardiography to diagnosis and management. Echocardiography 16:297-306, 1999

Non-Atherosclerosis MI

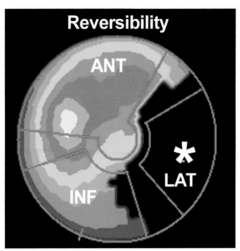

99m Technetium Sestamibi Bullseye projection showing a fixed (infarction) lateral hypoactivity (*) in left circum-flex coronary artery territory, in a young patient involved in a car accident.

Key Facts
- EKG and enzymes similar to typical acute myocardial infarction (MI)
- Younger patient population with less risk factors except for cigarette smoking
- 6% of acute myocardial infarction (AMI) have normal coronary arteries at autopsy

Imaging Findings
General Findings
- Diminished perfusion and function to the affected area
- Reduced regional perfusion, function and metabolism
Chest Radiography Findings
- Interstitial edema if heart failure ensues
2D Echocardiography Findings
- Altered ventricular function
Cardiac Scintigraphy Findings
- Reduced or absent tracer uptake
- No redistribution of thallium or re-injection uptake of Tc 99m
Ventricular Angiography Findings
- Reduced regional wall motion and ejection fraction
- Reduced wall thickening, or evident thinning (dyskinesis)
Coronary Angiography Findings
- Occluded coronary artery
- Patent but tightly stenotic coronary artery, or plaque disruption
MR Findings
- Reduced wall motion and ejection fraction on cine MR
- Delayed hyperenhancement

Non-Atherosclerosis MI

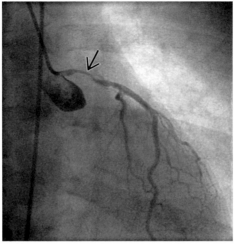

Right anterior oblique (RAO) cranial left coronary artery selective angiogram showing a radiation therapy induced severe left main (LM) stenosis (arrow), responsible for a large antero-lateral infarct, in a 42-year-old woman with a history of lymphoma treated by chest radiation.

Differential Diagnosis
<u>Coronary Artery Stenosis</u>
<u>Embolus</u>
- Nonbacterial thrombotic and infectious endocarditis
- Mural thrombi
- Prosthetic valves

<u>Vascular Inflammation</u>
- Syphilitis aortitis with ostial narrowing
- Coxsackie virus B
- Takayasu arteritis
- Radiation induced wall thickening
- Polyarteritis nodosa, systemic lupus erythematosus (SLE) and giant cell arteritis

<u>Chest Trauma</u>
<u>Cocaine Abuse</u>

Pathology
<u>General</u>
- Vascular occlusion and myocardial necrosis

Clinical Issues
<u>Presentation</u>
- Typical AMI presentation (see "Acute Myocardial Infarction") in younger aged population
- No history of angina, no prodrome prior to AMI

<u>Treatment & Prognosis</u>
- Standard therapy for AMI (see "Acute Myocardial Infarction")
- Greater survival than patients with AMI from atherosclerosis

Non-Atherosclerosis MI

Selected References
1.   Antman EM et al: Acute Myocardial Infarction In: Braundwald E. Heart Disease: A Textbook of Cardiovascular Medicine, 6th ed. W.B. Saunders Company, Philadelphia, 2001
2.   Topol EJ et al: Acute Myocardial Infarction. In: Topol EJ. Textbook of Cardiovascular Medicine, 6th ed. W.B. Lippincott Raven, Philadelphia, 395-436, 1998

Ischemic Cardiomyopathy

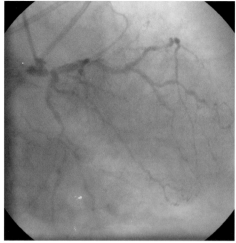

Right anterior oblique (RAO) caudal left coronary angiogram showing multiple coronary artery stenosis on left anterior descending (LAD) and left circumflex (coronary artery) (LCX) arteries, as well as their branches. Similar findings were depicted on the right coronary artery (RCA).

Key Facts
- Severe left ventricular (LV) dysfunction
- Multivessel coronary artery disease
- Global or regional LV dysfunction

Imaging Findings
General Findings
- Dilated hypokinetic left ventricle
- May have ischemic hypokinetic territory

Chest Radiography Findings
- Enlarged cardiac silhouette
- Often globular shaped heart
- May reveal evidence of heart failure
  - Kerley B lines, interstitial edema and vascular redistribution

Echocardiography Findings
- 2D echocardiography
  - Wall thinning and reduced ventricular function
  - Dilated mitral annulus
- Doppler echocardiography
  - Mitral regurgitation (MR) with papillary muscle dysfunction

Radionuclide Angiography Findings
- Reduced overall ejection fraction
- Global and regional myocardial dysfunction

Cardiac Scintigraphy Findings
- Reduced tracer uptake and wall thinning
- Increased chamber size
- Viable and ischemic regions

Ventricular Angiography Findings
- Reduced wall motion and ejection fraction, reduced wall thickening

Ischemic Cardiomyopathy

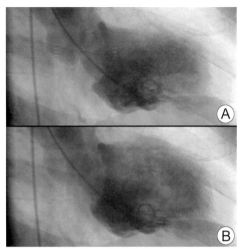

Left ventricle (LV) angiograms in systole (A) diastole (B) showing marked left ventricular dysfunction with reduced LV ejection fraction.

Coronary Angiography Findings
- Coronary stenoses and occlusions in several territories

MR Findings
- Reduced wall motion and ejection fraction on cine MR
- May have zones of infarction detected with delayed hyperenhancement

Differential Diagnosis
Coronary Artery Stenosis
Old Infarction
- Wall motion abnormalities
- Persistent hyperenhancement on MRI
- Absent tracer uptake on scintigraphy

Myocarditis
- Membrane integrity is compromised
- Occasionally require angiography for diagnosis
- If process is diffuse, differential diagnosis in the absence of shock makes diagnosis of myocarditis more secure

Idiopathic Dilated Cardiomyopathy
- Absent or insignificant coronary artery disease
  - Not always easy to determine significance
  - Coronary disease not necessarily reliably graded by severity of stenosis on coronary angiography
- Diagnosis of exclusion
- Genotyping may suggest heredofamilial illness

Pathology
General
- Myocardial necrosis, vascular occlusion
- Most often combined with ischemic or post-ischemic non-infarcted myocardium

Ischemic Cardiomyopathy

Clinical Issues

Presentation

- Chest pain: Substernal, pressing, occasionally radiating to the left arm
  - Typical features of myocardial infarction may precede development of ischemic cardiomyopathy
  - May be preceded by silent infarcts
  - Symptoms of heart failure, depending on state of compensation
- Symptoms associated with arrhythmias: Atrial or ventricular

Treatment & Prognosis

- Poor prognosis for 5-year survival; depends on
  - Ejection fraction
  - Functional status; poor class IV survival
  - Arrhythmias
- Therapy for acute myocardial infarction (MI) can preserve tissue and alter progression of disease
  - Thrombolysis, Percutaneous intervention
- Medical therapy
  - Diuretics to reduce symptoms and allow patients to tolerate other medications; optimum medical management in euvolemic patients
  - Reduce activity of renin-angiotensin-aldosterone system
    - ACE inhibitors in all patients without significant side effects
    - Angiotensin blockers (AT1 blockers); currently reserved for patients intolerant of ACE inhibitors
  - Beta blockers in all euvolemic patients without recent symptomatic heart failure or requirement for beta agonists
    - Conclusive data with carvedilol, metoprolol, and bisoprolol
    - Intolerance for heart failure decompensation or bradycardia
  - Digoxin: May reduce rate of hospitalization, no effect on mortality
  - Aspirin: Reduces risk of coronary thrombosis
  - Cholesterol lowering therapy: Statin therapy to reduce recurrent infarct
- Coronary revascularization (bypass surgery) can improve prognosis
  - Most reliable in patients with angina
  - Best data in patients with viable myocardium
    - PET: Level of perfusion adequate using NH3 or other perfusion tracer, or residual metabolic activity
    - Dobutamine echo: Improved function with low level dose
    - MRI: Absence of delayed hyperenhancement
  - Surgical risk is high; however, these patients derive the greatest benefit
- Implantable defibrillator (indications still under investigation)
  - Latest data supports implantation in patients with
    - Inducible or spontaneous arrhythmias
    - All patients with ejection fraction < 30% with ischemic etiology
- Transplantation
  - Intractable heart failure or arrhythmias
  - Benefit of revascularization expected to be minimal

Selected References
1. Gheorghiade M et al: Chronic heart failure in the United States: A manifestation of coronary artery disease. Circulation 97:282, 1998
2. Burch GE et al: Ischemic cardiomyopathy. Am Heart J 79:291, 1970

Subendocardial Myocardial Infarction

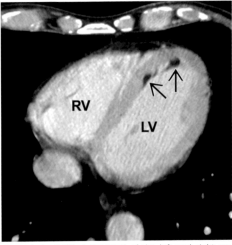

Contrast enhanced chest CT at the level of the left and right ventricle (RV). Subendocardial hypodense myocardium (arrows) at the level of the septum and the apico-septal left ventricle (LV), consistent with small infarcts.

Key Facts
- Most often diagnosed on the basis of EKG
- Confirmed by detection of markers in the serum
- Imaging may show thinning or partial thickness perfusion
  - Dependent on image resolution
  - Infarct detection may be compromised by partial volume effects

Imaging Findings
General Findings
- Diminished perfusion and function in the affected area
  - Functional impairment is limited if minimal thickness involved
- Imaging will not detect some nontransmural infarcts
Echocardiography Finding
- Reduced regional function
Radionuclide Angiography Finding
- Reduced regional function
Cardiac Scintigraphy Findings
- Using perfusion marker, reduced tracer uptake demonstrated
  - Usually apparent as wall thinning rather than dropout
Coronary Angiography Findings
- More commonly tightly stenosed coronary artery rather than occlusion
- Tight stenoses which become occluded more likely to cause nontransmural infarct than mild stenoses which occlude
  - Chronic flow reduction may be a stimulus for collateral formation
MR Findings
- Reduced wall motion
- Reduced wall thickening
- Increased signal intensity on T2 weighted imaging
- Reduced or delayed uptake of contrast agent on dynamic imaging

Subendocardial Myocardial Infarction

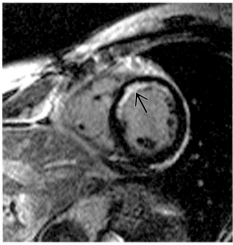

Late phase gadolinium enhanced gated MRI, in short axis. Subendocardial left ventricle (LV) hyperintense signal is noted (arrow), consistent with a left anterior descending (LAD) infarction.

- o Reduced signal enhancement with T1 weighted imaging using Gd agent
- Delayed hyperenhancement
  - o Likely will become the gold standard for detection and quantification
  - o The high resolution images enable clear partial thickness imaging

CT Findings
- Subendocardial non-enhancing segment of the left ventricle (LV)

Differential Diagnosis
Coronary Artery Stenosis
Old Infarction with Thinned Myocardium
- Scintigraphy is a poor discriminating technique
- Persistent hyperenhancement on MRI cannot discriminate old from new infarct
  - o Will demonstrate infarct rather than thinning

Myocarditis
- Patchy nature of disease may appear as nontransmural infarct
  - o Serum markers and wall motion assessment will not adequately discriminate this diagnoses from infarction
  - o Coronary angiography is essential

Pathology
General
- Myocardial necrosis
  - o Coagulation necrosis
  - o Contraction band necrosis
  - o Intramyocardial hemorrhage
- Vascular occlusion
- Result of early reperfusion before wavefront of infarction can extend transmurally

Subendocardial Myocardial Infarction

Clinical Issues

<u>Presentation</u>
- Chest pain; clinical picture of acute myocardial infarction (MI)
- Clinically determined by absence of Q wave on EKG, with serum marker of myocardial infarction (MI) and appropriate clinical presentation
  - o Poor discrimination from transmural MI
- More commonly seen without ST elevation on presentation EKG
  - o Natural history of MI not especially predictable on the basis of presenting EKG
- Not uncommonly result of early reperfusion; prevent transmural extension
  - o Thrombolysis
  - o Percutaneous intervention
- May be associated with lethal arrhythmias, similar to transmural MI
- Wall thickening may be maintained
  - o Result of varied orientation of myofibrils with wall thickness
  - o Loss of oblique subendocardial fibers will not necessarily cause loss of normal thickening

<u>Treatment & Prognosis</u>
- Medical therapy; thrombolysis or early mechanical reperfusion can prevent progression of transmural infarct; salvage outer myocardial layers
  - o Early reperfusion may prevent infarction altogether
- Acute percutaneous intervention to restore flow
  - o Best done within the first 3 hours
  - o Optimally done with stent implantation and antiplatelet therapy with Gp IIb/IIIa inhibitor
- Prognosis depends on extent of infarction and degree and location of coronary disease
- Nontransmural infarcts associated with
  - o Better prognosis
  - o Less infarct expansion
  - o Decreased risk of cardiac rupture
  - o Mural thrombosis
  - o LV aneurysm

Selected References
1. Weissman HF et al: Effect of extent of transmurality on infarct expansion. Clin Res 32:477A, 1984
2. Reimer KA et al: The wavefront phenomenon of myocardial cell death: Transmural progression of necrosis within the framework of ischemic bed size (myocardium at risk) and collateral flow. Lab Invest 40:633, 1979

Post Infarction LV Aneurysm

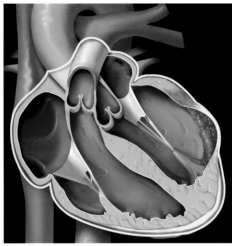

Large transmural infarct of the antero-lateral left ventricle (LV), resulting in a thin walled outpouching. Thrombus is overlying the endocardial aspect of the aneurysm.

Key Facts
- More common with left anterior descending (LAD) disease
- Can lead to intractable heart failure
- Indicates poor prognosis
- Risk of systemic emboli

Imaging Findings
General Findings
- Thinned myocardium
- Broad neck
- Dyskinesis, paradoxical motion

Chest Radiography Findings
- Enlarged cardiac silhouette
- Occasionally can identify aneurysm as demarcated outpouching
- Calcified left ventricle (LV) aneurysm may be identified

Echocardiography Findings
- Excellent method to identify aneurysm
- Clear demonstration of paradoxical motion
- Doppler evidence of flow into the aneurysm
- Can demonstrate thrombus in the aneurysm
- Common to find "smoke" in aneurysm, suggesting slow flow and likelihood of thrombus formation

Radionuclide Scintigraphy Findings
- Paradoxical motion
- Ventricular enlargement

MR Findings
- Cine imaging reveals paradoxical motion
- Increased signal intensity; reduced flow velocity in the aneurysm attenuates intravoxel phase dispersion

Post Infarction LV Aneurysm

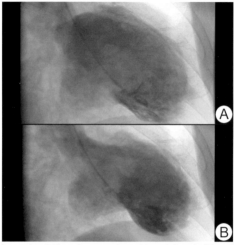

Selective left ventricle (LV) angiograms showed in end diastole (A) and end systole (B) demonstrating a post myocardial infarction (MI) large LV aneurysm, with paradoxical motion during systole, where its apical portion is enlarged.

- Thinned left ventricular wall is apparent
- Frequent filling defect consistent with mural thrombus

CT Findings
- Dynamics of aneurysm apparent with fast gated imaging
- Thinned left ventricular wall is apparent
- Frequent filling defect consistent with mural thrombus

Catheterization Findings
- Most often coronary occlusion in vessel supplying infarcted territory
- More common with occlusion of LAD than other vessels
- Typically absent coronary collaterals
- Aneurysm apparent on ventriculogram

Differential Diagnosis
Pseudoaneurysm
- Narrow neck
- Contained rupture, may demonstrate some contrast in the pericardial space

Pathology
General
- Transmural infarct
- Mixture of fibrous tissue, infarcted and non-infarcted myocardium
- Frequently with evidence of pericarditis; inflamed or adherent pericardium
- Longstanding aneurysms may calcify
- More common in the anterior wall or apex

Clinical Issues
Presentation
- Persistent ST elevation after myocardial infarction (MI); may be more representative of large infarct

Post Infarction LV Aneurysm

- Palpable heave on physical exam; occasionally with paradoxical impulse
- Frequently asymptomatic
- Heart failure
- Stroke or peripheral embolus

Natural History
- Less than 10% of patients with acute myocardial infarction (AMI)
- Mostly anterior or anterior-apical wall
- Rarely rupture
- Calcify over several years
- May continue to expand, though rare
- Mortality 6x higher than in patients without aneurysms

Treatment
- Blood pressure control is essential
- ACE inhibitor recommended in all patients after MI
  - Reduce infarct expansion
- Beta blockers to control heart rate response
- Anticoagulants, warfarin
  - 3-6 months after infarct
  - Some physicians prolong therapy if thrombus apparent on echo
    - Especially if mobile, sessile, or protruding into cavity
- Aneurysmectomy
  - Indications: Angina, heart failure, or arrhythmias that are intractable despite optimal medical therapy
  - Must have sufficient functional myocardium remaining to warrant risk of surgery
  - Best done with well-defined neck to aneurysm

Selected References
1. Antman EM et al: Acute Myocardial Infarction. In: Braundwald E. Heart Disease: A Textbook of Cardiovascular Medicine. 6th ed. W.B. Saunders Company, Philadelphia, 2001
2. Ha JW et al: Left ventricular aneurysm after myocardial infarction. Clin Cardiol 21:917, 1998
3. Meizlish JL et al: Functional left ventricular aneurysm formation after acute anterior myocardial infarction: Incidence, natural history, and prognostic implications. N Engl J 311:1001, 1984

Left Ventricular Free Wall Rupture

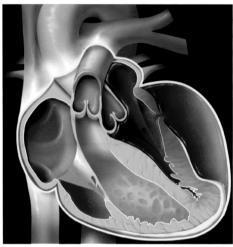

Left ventricle (LV) free wall infarction with myocardial rupture. Pericardial blood effusion with LV tamponade.

Key Facts
- Left ventricular (LV) wall rupture in acute myocardial infarction (MI) with sudden hemodynamic deterioration
- Tamponade physiology
- Hemopericardium: Fibrinous pericardial effusion and occasional clots on echo, blood apparent on CT, high T2 on MRI
- Emergent surgery and early recognition is critical

Imaging Findings
<u>General Features</u>
- Pericardial effusion
- Evidence of hemopericardium

<u>Chest Radiography Findings</u>
- Enlarged cardiac silhouette
- Flask-shaped heart, typical of pericardial effusion
- Absence of signs of heart failure

<u>Echocardiography Findings</u>
- 2D echocardiography
  - Pericardial effusion; may not be large noting acute accumulation
  - May show evidence of thrombi or fibrinous material in pericardial fluid
  - In subacute rupture, pseudoaneurysm may be apparent with thrombus and narrow communication
  - Tamponade physiology, diastolic right ventricle (RV) or right atrium (RA) collapse
  - Shows associated myocardial pathology: Recent MI with akinesis or dyskinesis, or evidence of trauma
- Doppler Echocardiography
  - Enhanced respiratory phasic variation characteristic of tamponade
  - May be able to demonstrate communication between left ventricle (LV) and pericardium (or pseudoaneurysm)

Left Ventricular Free Wall Rupture

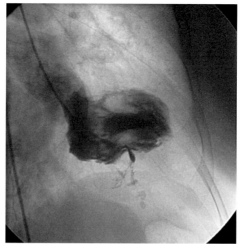

Selective LV angiogram indicating an inferior LV wall rupture, with contrast extravasation into the pericardium, secondary to a transmural infarct.

Left Ventricular Angiography Findings
- Delineation of region of communication between LV and pericardial space
- If thrombus restricts communication, contrast penetration will be less helpful
- Identifies region of reduced wall motion

MR Findings
- Pericardial effusion, suggestion of hemopericardium with variable intensity suggesting thrombi, and signal intensity matching blood
- Contrast may demonstrate communication of LV with pericardial space
- Wall motion abnormalities or evidence of trauma
- Communication may be apparent between LV and pericardial space

CT Findings
- Attenuation in the pericardial space matches blood
- Wall motion abnormalities or evidence of trauma
- Communication may be apparent between LV and pericardial space

Differential Diagnosis

Acute Myocardial Rupture (MR), Papillary Muscle Rupture
- Heart failure apparent
- Echo evidence of flail leaflet
- No pericardial effusion or tamponade

Ventricular Septal Rupture
- Harsh continuous murmur with thrill on examination
- Absence of pericardial effusion

Marked Systolic Dysfunction with Extension of Myocardial Infarction
- Reduced ejection fraction
- Absence of other mechanical defects cited above

Extension of Ascending Aortic Dissection into the Pericardium
- Echo, MR and CT will demonstrate the dissection associated with hemopericardium

Left Ventricular Free Wall Rupture

Pathology

General
- Infarction in the absence of collaterals

Gross Pathologic, Surgical Features
- Stuttering progressive process of intramural infiltrating hemorrhage
- Noted approximately equally in anterior, posterior, and lateral distributions
- 3 typical variants
  - Slit like: Early infarct
    - Seen within the first 12 hrs
    - Associated with delayed thrombolysis (> 14 hrs after infarction)
  - Erosion at the borders of the infarct; extension of infarct, intermediate in timing
  - Expansion of the infarct; large infarction, late appearing
- Pseudoaneurysm; subacute contained rupture with thrombus in the pericardial space

Clinical Issues

Presentation
- Occurs early (< 24 hrs), and late (4-7 days) post infarction
  - Incidence of 6.2% in a study of 1,457 patients
- Recurrent chest pain
- Repetitive emesis, restlessness and agitation
- Sudden sometimes transient episode of hypotension and bradycardia
- Persistent tachycardia without other obvious cause
- Most common: First MI, elderly (age > 60), women
  - Other risks: Hypertension, lack of collaterals, transmural MI, corticosteroids or nonsteroidal antiinflammatories, and thrombolytic therapy > 14 hrs after onset of infarction

Natural History
- High mortality in the absence of prompt treatment

Treatment & Prognosis
- Emergent surgical repair; high long-term survival if surgery is successful
- Surgery should be arranged expeditiously once the diagnosis is made
  - Clinical suspicion is most important in making a diagnosis
  - Hemodynamic compromise in the setting of an acute MI, with a new pericardial effusion and tamponade physiology indicates a high likelihood of rupture
- Pericardiocentesis will confirm the presence of hemopericardium; however, it can be DANGEROUS in the setting of subacute LV rupture and increase the likelihood of further LV leakage.

Selected References
1. Becker RC et al: A composite view of cardiac rupture in the United States national registry of myocardial infarction. J Am Coll Cardiol 27:1321-26, 1996
2. Pollak H et al: Frequency of left ventricular free wall rupture complicating acute myocardial infarction since the advent of thrombolysis. Am J Cardiol 74:184-6, 1994
3. Nakamura F et al: Cardiac free wall rupture in acute myocardial infarction: Ameliorative effect of coronary reperfusion. Clin Cardiol 15:244-50, 1992

Ventricular Septal Rupture

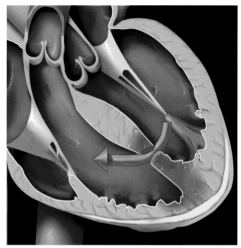

Ventricular septal defect (VSD) due to infarction will induce a left to right shunt across the septum with associated right ventricular volume overload enlargement.

Key Facts
- Complication of anterior or inferior wall infarction
- New ventricular septal defect (VSD) apparent on echo
- Right ventricular volume overload
- A mechanical cause of hemodynamic collapse post-myocardial infarction (MI)
- Requires prompt surgical treatment

Imaging Findings

General Features
- Right ventricular enlargement
- Left to right shunt across the ventricular septum
- Size of infarct in part determines prognosis

Chest Radiography Findings
- Right ventricle (RV) enlargement
- Pulmonary congestion

Echocardiography Findings
- 2D echocardiography
  - RV enlargement
  - Ventricular septal defect (VSD)
  - Wall motion abnormalities corresponding to the infarction
- Doppler echocardiography
  - Demonstration of a shunt across the ventricular septum
  - Bubble contrast is rarely necessary
- Transesophageal echocardiography
  - Used more commonly in seriously ill patients in the ICU or operating room

Left Ventricular Angiography Findings
- Easy demonstration of the VSD with left ventricular injection
  - Rapid appearance of contrast in the right ventricle

Ventricular Septal Rupture

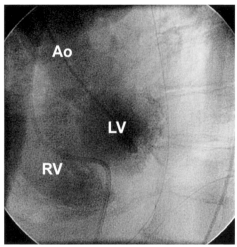

Left anterior oblique (LAO) caudal left ventricle (LV) selective angiogram during systole, showing large opacification of the right ventricle (RV), secondary to a septal rupture after myocardial infarction (MI).

- Permits evaluation of coronary anatomy to guide possible coronary bypass during VSD repair

<u>Pulmonary Artery Catheterization Findings</u>
- Demonstrate an oxygen step up in the right ventricle (RV) and pulmonary artery (PA)
  - o Important to sample from the proximal PA to avoid sampling regurgitant blood associated with cases of severe mitral regurgitation
  - o Rarely needed for diagnosis with adequate echocardiogram

<u>MR Findings</u>
- Angiographic sequence (short TR short TE) sequence can demonstrate the shunt and, if a jet results across the VSD, will show a flow void in the RV
- Right ventricular enlargement
- Infarct detection with contrast induced delayed hyperenhancement

Differential Diagnosis
<u>Acute Mitral Regurgitation</u>
- Papillary muscle infarction, or chordal rupture
- MR is easily distinguished from a VSD by echocardiography or ventriculography

<u>Cardiogenic Shock</u>
- Marked reduction in cardiac function by any modality

Pathology
<u>General</u>
- Necrosis of the ventricular septum
  - o Direct communication across the septum, usually at the ventricular apex for anterior infarction
  - o Complex serpiginous hemorrhagic communication across the inferobasal septum more commonly associated with inferior MI

Ventricular Septal Rupture

  o Anterior and anterolateral infarcts are slightly more common than inferior infarcts

Clinical Issues
Presentation
- Recurrent chest pain after an infarction
- More common with first infarcts, occurs in 1-3% of MIs
- Can occur within the first 24 hrs, or first week
- Evidence of high right sided pressure out of proportion to the extent of pulmonary congestion
- New holosystolic murmur with a thrill over the left sternal border

Natural History
- Untreated: Symptomatic patients have a high mortality

Treatment & Prognosis
- Medical therapy to reduce afterload using intra-aortic balloon
- Urgent cardiac catheterization to define coronary anatomy for possible bypass and confirm the diagnosis
  o Especially important to define mitral valve competence
- Pericardial patch with or without infarct resection
- Higher mortality when inferior MI and RV infarction as compared to anterior MI

Selected References
1. Held AC et al: Rupture of the interventricular septum complicating acute myocardial infarction: A multicenter analysis of clinical findings and outcome. Am Heart J 116:1330–6, 1988
2. Radford MJ et al: Ventricular septal rupture: A review of clinical and physiologic features and an analysis of survival. Circulation 64:545–53, 1981

Left Ventricular Thrombus

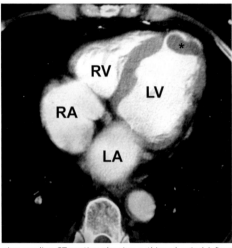

4-chamber view cardiac CT section showing a thinned apical left ventricle (LV) myocardium with an attached non-enhanced mass (*) consistent with a post myocardial infarction (MI) thrombus.

Key Facts
- Frequent finding in anterior myocardial infarction (MI), and more commonly with dyskinetic segments
- Associated with blood stasis, increased coagulation, endothelial injury
- Risk for thromboembolism

Imaging Findings
General Features
- Found in the setting of reduced wall motion
  - Post MI
  - Cardiomyopathy
- May have an irregular border
- Depending on the imaging modality, must be distinguished from the neighboring myocardium
- Size and shape of the thrombus can have prognostic significance

Echocardiography Findings
- 2D echocardiography
  - 70-80% sensitivity, 90-95% specificity
  - More echodense than neighboring myocardium
  - Laminated or pedunculated
  - Occasionally with fibrinous attachments
  - Associated with wall motion abnormalities and aneurysm formation
  - Shaggy or mobile thrombi are more likely to embolize
- Doppler echocardiography
  - Abnormal flow patterns neighboring thrombus representing stasis

Left Ventricular Angiography Findings
- Space-occupying lesion in area of reduced wall motion
- Can demonstrate dye penetration in border zone between thrombus and myocardium

Left Ventricular Thrombus

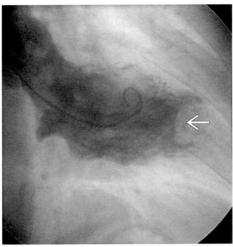

Selective LV angiogram, showing a filling defect of the apex, (arrow) suggesting a thrombus.

MR Findings
- Region of differential intensity which depends on the age of the thrombus
  - With T2-weighted imaging can change from high intensity to low as thrombus matures
  - Can also be seen as very short T1WI material as high spin iron appears during thrombus metabolism

Differential Diagnosis
Papillary Muscles
- Move concordant with valve motion
False Tendons
- Trabeculations
Technical Artifacts
- Not apparent on multiple views
- Not associated with stasis
Bicuspid Valve
- Thickening leaflets produces incomplete closure and/or prolapse
Cardiac Tumors (Benign and Malignant)

Pathology
General
- Can be red or mixed red and white thrombus
- Thrombus may form on the surface of a tumor making diagnosis more problematic
Myocardium
- Associated with
  - Myocardial infarction
  - Ventricular aneurysm
  - Cardiomyopathy

Left Ventricular Thrombus

Clinical Issues

<u>Presentation</u>
- Recent MI or diagnosis of cardiomyopathy

<u>Natural History</u>
- Found in 30-40% with anterior MI, but < 5% with inferior MI
- 55-85% of thrombi were shown to resolve in a 3 year period without treatment

<u>Treatment & Prognosis</u>
- Warfarin anticoagulation
  - o Observational studies suggest some benefit in prevention of thromboembolism
    - In one study 90% of thrombi resolved in 6 months without any emboli
  - o Current ACC/AHA recommendations **do not support** the use of prolonged anticoagulation in the absence of prospective studies
  - o Depending on the characteristics of the thrombus, 3 months of anticoagulation may be a reasonable compromise

Selected References
1. Kontny F et al: Left ventricular thrombus formation and resolution in acute myocardial infarction. Int J Cardiol 66(2):169-74, 1998
2. Kouvaras G et al: The effects of long tern anti-thrombotic treatment on left ventricular thrombi in patients after an acute myocardial infarction. Am Heart J 119:73-7, 1990
3. Weintraub WS et al: Decision analysis concerning the application of echocardiography to the diagnosis and treatment of mural thrombi after anterior wall acute myocardial infarction. Am J Cardiol 64:708-16, 1989

Post Angioplasty Restenosis

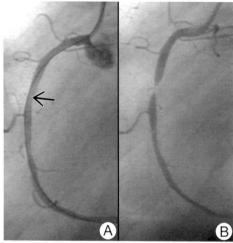

(A) Final right coronary angiogram after percutaneous transluminal coronary angioplasty (PTCA) (arrow), showing good result. (B) Same patient 6 months later. A severe restenosis is demonstrated. Successful stent implantation was then performed.

Key Facts
- Balloon angioplasty is associated with vascular injury or dissection
- Healing frequently results in tissue ingrowth and restenosis
- Post angioplasty lumen size: Prognostic indicator of clinical restenosis

Imaging Findings
General Findings
- Varied characteristics of stenotic lesion
  - Concentric or eccentric
  - Smooth or rough

Catheterization Findings
- Diffuse or focal lesion development
- May show evidence of dissection

CT, MR Findings
- Potential imaging by MRI or CT, though no study yet completed

Differential Diagnosis
Coronary Artery Stenosis
- New coronary stenosis on a non previously treated segment

Pathology
General
- Elastic recoil
- Reduction in area delimited by external and internal elastic laminae
- Neointimal growth may play a lesser role than initially assumed

Clinical Issues
Presentation
- Most often asymptomatic restenosis
- Commonly occurs within 6 months of the procedure

Post Angioplasty Restenosis

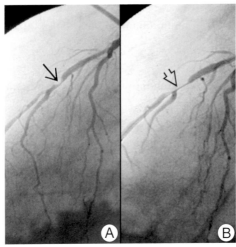

(A) Original mid left anterior descending (LAD) stenosis (arrow), successfully treated with PTCA. (B) Same patient 4 months later. A severe restenosis is depicted (open arrow). Stent implantation was performed.

- Estimated 30-50% restenosis rate
- Can present with typical ischemic symptoms
  - Recurrent angina
  - Acute myocardial infarction (MI)
  - Sudden onset heart failure
- Greater incidence after treatment of total occlusion, small vessels, long lesions, thrombus, complicated dissections
- Worse outcome in diabetics, heart failure, old age, smokers

Prevention
- Aspirin (indefinitely)
- Gp IIb/IIIa inhibitor periprocedure
- Careful balloon sizing
- Avoidance of over expansion
- Stent placement reduced restenosis by 30-50%

Treatment
- Repeat balloon angioplasty
- Stent placement
  - Preferred treatment in vessels > 2.5 mm
- Rotational atherectomy
- Coronary bypass for severe stenoses not amenable to percutaneous treatment, or patients with multivessel disease

Selected References
1. Landzberg BR et al: Pathophysiology and pharmacologic approaches for prevention of coronary artery restenosis following coronary artery balloon angioplasty and related procedures. Prog Cardiovasc Disease 39:361, 1997
2. Bittl JA: Medical progress: Advances in coronary angioplasty. N Engl J Med 335:1290-302, 1996

Post Stent Restenosis

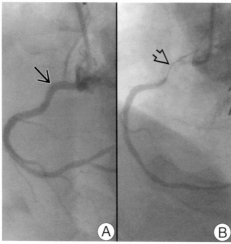

(A) Excellent result after stenting (arrow) of the ostial and proximal right coronary artery (RCA). (B) Severe restenosis (open arrow) inside the RCA stent after 4 months.

Key Facts
- Neointimal proliferation
- Less common than with simple balloon angioplasty
- May appear anywhere along the stent, including the edges

Imaging Findings
General Features
- Potential imaging by MRI or CT, though stent artifact remains a problem

Catheterization Findings
- In most cases stent has low to moderate visibility
- Restenosis at stent edges "candy wrapper lesions" with some radiation treated stents
- Subacute thrombosis, edge dissection

Differential Diagnosis
Coronary Artery Stenosis
- New coronary stenosis on a non previously stented segment

Pathology
General
- Neointimal proliferation
- More cellular and proliferative, and less of a thrombotic response than after simple balloon angioplasty

Clinical Issues
Presentation
- Most often asymptomatic restenosis within 6-12 months
- 15-20% restenosis depending on stent type, length, diameter, and post deployment minimal luminal diameter
- Recurrent angina

Post Stent Restenosis

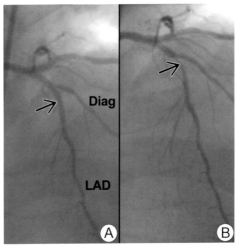

(A) Successful stent implantation in the mid left anterior descending (LAD) (arrow), just after the origin of a large diagonal branch. (B) Severe restenosis inside the LAD stent (arrow), 7 months later.

- Acute myocardial infarction (MI)
- Sudden onset heart failure

Prevention

- Aspirin (indefinitely) and clopidogrel (4 weeks)
- Gp IIb/IIIa inhibitor periprocedure
- Adequate deployment with full stent expansion and contact
  - Intravascular ultrasound guidance used by some practitioners
- Avoidance of over expansion at stent edges
- Novel therapies; marked reduction in restenosis
  - Radiation treatment; gamma or beta emitters; 2/3 reduction in target lesion revascularization
  - Sirolimus or tacrolimus treated "coated" stents

Treatment

- Balloon angioplasty
- Rotational atherectomy
- Excimer laser ablation
- Repeat stenting
- 30% recurrence without novel therapies (see above)
- Benefit of repeat stenting now open to question
- Coronary bypass for severe stenoses not amenable to percutaneous treatment

Selected References

1. Mehran R et al: Treatment of focal in-stent restenosis with balloon angioplasty alone versus stenting: Short- and long-term results. Am Heart J 141:610–4, 2001
2. Goldberg SL et al: Rotational atherectomy or balloon angioplasty in the treatment of intra-stent restenosis: BARASTER multicenter registry. Catheter Cardiovasc Interv 51:407–13, 2000
3. Teirstein PS et al: Catheter-based radiotherapy to inhibit restenosis after coronary stenting. N Engl J Med 336:1697–703, 1997

Post CABG Thrombosis

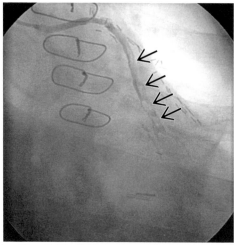

Right anterior oblique (RAO) selective angiogram of a coronary artery bypass graft (CABG), showing several filling defects (arrows) inside the vein graft, corresponding to thrombi.

Key Facts
- Saphenous vein thrombosis: Early cause of graft failure
- ~ 10% of coronary artery bypass graft (CABG) occluded during the first month post surgery

Imaging Findings
General Features
- Early occlusion of graft
- Abnormal perfusion and function in region subtended by graft

Catheterization Findings
- Demonstrates graft occlusion
- Abnormal wall motion on ventriculogram

Nuclear Cardiology Findings
- Thallium or technetium imaging
  - Reduced tracer uptake in ischemic

MRA and CTA Findings
- Demonstrates occlusion of graft

Differential Diagnosis
Coronary Artery Stenosis
- New stenosis on native coronary arteries

CABG Atherosclerosis (Stenosis)
Perioperative Infarction
- Especially in left main stenosis and triple vessel disease

Pathology
General
- Loss of endothelium with accumulation of fibrin
- Adherence of platelets and white blood cells
- Thrombus occluding vessel lumen especially at sites of anastomosis

Post CABG Thrombosis

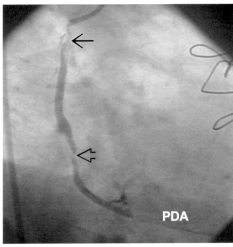

Selective angiogram of a venous graft to the posterior descending artery (PDA). Proximal thrombosis (arrow) and a stenosis (open arrow) of the graft are depicted.

Clinical Issues

<u>Presentation</u>
- Range from no symptoms to recurrent angina and infarction

<u>Prevention</u>
- Use of arterial conduits including internal mammary and radial arteries
- Aggressive antiplatelet therapies

<u>Treatment</u>
- Standard treatment for ischemia
  - See "Coronary Artery Stenosis"
  - See "Acute Myocardial Infarction"

Selected References
1. Antman EM et al: Acute Myocardial Infarction In: Braundwald E. Heart Disease: A Textbook of Cardiovascular Medicine. 6th ed W.B. Saunders Company, Philadelphia, 2001
2. Motwani JG et al: Aortocoronary saphenous vein graft disease: Pathogenesis, predisposition and prevention. Circulation 97:916-31, 1998

Post CABG Atherosclerosis

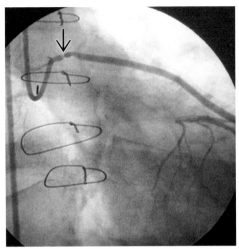

Selective vein graft angiogram to left anterior descending (LAD) showing a severe proximal stenosis (arrow). Successful stent implantation was achieved.

Key Facts
- Significant stenosis or occlusion of bypass graft
- Accelerated form of atherosclerosis
- By 10 years ~ 50% of grafts are occluded
- Late graft thrombosis occurs with or without symptoms

Imaging Findings
General Features
- Severe stenosis or occlusion of graft
- Abnormal perfusion and function in region subtended by graft

Catheterization Findings
- Demonstrates degree of luminal stenosis or occlusion
- Abnormal wall motion on ventriculogram

Nuclear Cardiology Findings
- Thallium or technetium imaging
  - Reduced tracer uptake in ischemic area (see "Coronary Artery Stenosis")

MRA and CTA Findings
- Demonstrates severe stenosis and occlusion of graft

Differential Diagnosis
Coronary Artery Stenosis

Pathology
General
- Neointimal hyperplasia
- Proliferation of smooth muscle cells and extracellular matrix
- Proliferation throughout the length of the graft with focal areas of stenosis

Post CABG Atherosclerosis

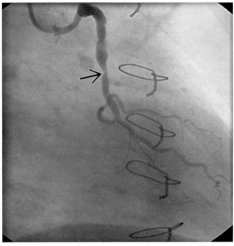

Selective angiogram of a venous coronary artery bypass graft (CABG) to a marginal branch of the left circumflex (LCX), showing irregular aspect of the wall corresponding to atherosclerosis, with a 60% stenosis in its mid portion (arrow).

- Acute thrombosis found in approximately 70% of patients undergoing re-operation

Clinical Issues

Presentation
- Angina recurs in 15-20% of patients during the first year post op with an additional ~ 4% per year
- Approximately 25 of patients require re-operation in 10 years

Prevention
- Use of arterial conduits including internal mammary which is essentially immune to the development of intimal hyperplasia
- Intensive risk factor modification: Especially aggressive lipid-lowering and antiplatelet therapies

Treatment
- Standard treatment for ischemia or infarction

Prognosis
- Coronary artery bypass graft (CABG) re-operation carries a higher mortality ~ 3-7%

Selected References
1. Antman EM et al: Acute Myocardial Infarction In: Braundwald E. Heart Disease: A Textbook of Cardiovascular Medicine. 6th ed. W.B. Saunders Company, Philadelphia, 2001
2. Motwani JG et al: Aortocoronary saphenous vein graph disease: Pathogenesis, predisposition and prevention. Circulation 97:916-31, 1998

PocketRadiologist™
Cardiac
Top 100 Diagnoses

HEART FAILURE

Right Heart Failure

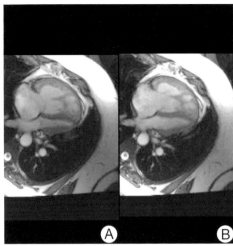

Right heart failure. (A) Systolic and (B) diastolic phase cine FIESTA images demonstrate marked enlargement of the right ventricle with global hypokinesis. Right ventricular ejection fraction was 18%.

Key Facts
- Chest radiograph classically demonstrates right sided cardiomegaly and elevated central venous volume
- Most common cause is left heart failure
- Cor Pulmonale = right heart failure due to pulmonary disease
- Associated with lower extremity edema, ascites, weight gain

Imaging Findings
Chest Radiography Findings
- Right-sided cardiomegaly
- Increased central venous volume (large azygous vein)

CT Findings
- Same

Echocardiography Findings
- Right ventricle (RV) function often difficult to assess on echo due to limited acoustic window
- RV Systolic dysfunction
- Decreased RV outflow tract acceleration time
- Tricuspid regurgitation
- Pulmonary regurgitation
- Dilated inferior vena cava (IVC) and hepatic veins

MR Findings
- MRI better for assessing RV functional parameters than echocardiography
- May be decreased ejection fraction from systolic dysfunction or decreased compliance from diastolic dysfunction
- Short-access cine-gradient echo imaging optimal method for assessing right ventricular mass and thickness (now SSFP: True FISP, FIESTA, balanced FE)
- Temporal resolution should be 25-40 m/sec in order to accurately assess systole and diastole time points

Right Heart Failure

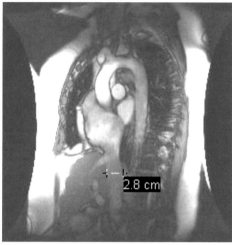

Right heart failure. Oblique sagittal view for same patient as prior image demonstrates marked enlargement of the IVC and hepatic veins, indicating elevated right-sided pressures. IVC measurement of 2.8 cm without respiratory phasic variation suggests right atrial pressure exceeding 20 mmHg.

- Normal RV functional parameters
  - RV end-diastolic volume 138 +/- 40 ml
  - RV end-systolic volume 54 +/- 21 ml
  - RV free wall mass 46 +/- 11 gm (26 +/- 5 gm/m^2)
  - RV ejection fraction (%) = 61 +/- 7
  - RV stroke volume = 84 +/- 24 ml (46 +/- 8 ml/m^2)
- Right atrial pressure ($P_{right\ atrium}$) estimated by size of IVC
  - Small (< 1.5 cm) 0-5 mmHg
  - Normal (1.5-2.5 cm) 5-15 mmHg
  - Dilated (> 2.5 cm) 15-20 mmHg
  - Dilated, enlarged hepatic veins > 20 mmHg

Differential Diagnosis
Non-Cardiogenic Edema
- Endstage liver disease with ascites and pleural effusions
- Renal disease

Isolated Left Heart Failure
- Typically pulmonary symptoms predominate

Pathology
General
- Typically pattern is chronic left ventricular function resulting in right heart failure from chronic overload
- Etiology-Pathogenesis
  - Left heart failure
  - Pulmonic stenosis
  - Shunts
  - Tricuspid valve disease
- Epidemiology

- o Very common result of left heart failure
- o Major source of morbidity and mortality in the United States

Gross Pathologic, Surgical Features
- Often dilated/hypertrophied right ventricle
- May see hypertrophied right atrium

Staging or Grading Criteria
- Class I: No limitation during ordinary activity
- Class II: Slight limitation by shortness of breath and/or fatigue during moderate exertion or stress
- Class III: Symptoms with minimal exertion that interfere with normal daily activity
- Class IV: Inability to carry out any physical activity; these patients typically have marked neurohumoral activation, muscle wasting, and reduced peak oxygen consumption

Clinical Issues

Presentation
- Lower extremity edema
- Ascites
- Weight gain
- Likely concomitant pulmonary symptoms

Treatment
- Diuretics
- Inotropics agents
- ACE inhibitors
- Beta blockers
- Treat underlying coronary disease

Prognosis
- Depends on NYHA Class
- Often more difficult to treat secondary to volume overload

Selected References
1. Braunwald E et al: Heart Disease: A Textbook of Cardiovascular Medicine. 6th Ed. W.B. Saunders Co., Philadelphia, 1751-83, 2001
2. Goldman L et al: Cecil Textbook of Medicine. 21st Ed. W.B. Saunders Co., Philadelphia, 207-26, 2000
3. Murray JF et al: Textbook of Respiratory Medicine. 3rd Ed. W.B. Saunders Co., Philadelphia, 2247-65, 2000

Left Heart Failure

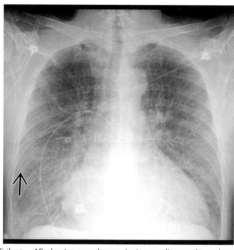

Left heart failure. AP chest x-ray demonstrates cardiomegaly, pulmonary venous hypertension, edema, and Kerley B lines (arrow), indicating left heart failure.

Key Facts
- Synonym: Congestive heart failure (CHF)
- Definition
  - Systolic dysfunction refers to a decrease in myocardial contractility
  - With pure diastolic heart failure, left ventricular end–systolic volume and stroke volume are preserved; there is, however, an abnormal decrease in left ventricular diastolic distensibility
  - Chest radiograph demonstrates enlarged cardiac silhouette with pulmonary edema and possibly pleural effusions

Imaging Findings
<u>Chest Radiography Finding</u>
- Cardiomegaly, pulmonary edema, pleural fluid
<u>CT Finding</u>
- Cardiomegaly, vascular redistribution, pleural fluid
<u>Echocardiography Findings</u>
- Variable depending on etiology
- Decreased ejection fraction with systolic dysfunction
- Decreased compliance with diastolic dysfunction
<u>MR Findings</u>
- Functional findings similar to echocardiography, but MRI more precise in quantifying myocardial functional parameters (i.e., stroke volume, ejection fraction)
- Delayed contrast-enhanced MRI may also be used to identify viable and non-viable myocardial tissue
- Viability on MRI may be used to predict response to beta-blocker therapy

Differential Diagnosis
<u>Etiology of Left Heart Failure</u>
- Ischemic
- Restrictive

Left Heart Failure

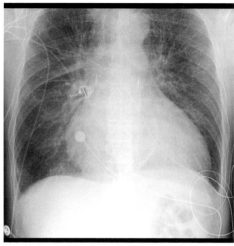

Resolved left heart failure. AP chest x-ray from same patient demonstrates persistent cardiomegaly but interval resolution of edema following treatment with diuretics.

- Constrictive
- Infiltrative disease

Pneumonia
- Atypical pneumonia may have diffuse air space disease/interstitial markings on chest radiograph

Pericardial Effusion
- Enlarged cardiac silhouette on chest radiograph

Pathology

General
- Genetics: Some component of inheritance for dilated cardiomyopathy and Idiopathic hypertrophic subaortic stenosis (IHSS) leading to left heart failure
- Etiology-Pathogenesis
  - The three major determinants of the left ventricular forward stroke volume/performance are the preload, myocardial contractility, and the afterload
  - The left atrium appears to adapt to left ventricular dysfunction in patients with CHF
- Epidemiology
  - One of the leading causes of death in the United States

Gross Pathologic, Surgical Features
- Often areas of infarcted myocardium in systolic dysfunction
- Myocyte hypertrophy vs. chamber enlargement

Microscopic Features
- Infarcted areas of myocardium in ischemic heart failure
- Infiltrating diseases in restrictive cardiomyopathy

Grading Criteria: New York Heart Association (NYHA) Classification
- Class I: No limitation during ordinary activity

- Class II: Slight limitation by shortness of breath and/or fatigue during moderate exertion or stress
- Class III: Symptoms with minimal exertion that interfere with normal daily activity
- Class IV: Inability to carry out any physical activity; these patients typically have marked neurohumoral activation, muscle wasting, and reduced peak oxygen consumption

Clinical Issues

Presentation
- Shortness of breath, dyspnea on exertion, orthopnea

Natural History
- Depending on NYHA Class

Treatment
- Diuretics
- Inotropics agents
- ACE inhibitors
- Beta blockers
- Treat underlying coronary disease

Prognosis
- Depends on NYHA Class
- Prognosis worsens with increasing NYHA class

Selected References
1. Braunwald E et al: Heart Disease: A Textbook of Cardiovascular Medicine. 6th Ed. W.B. Saunders Co., 1751-83, 2001
2. Goldman L et al: Cecil Textbook of Medicine. 21st Ed. W.B. Saunders Co., 207-26, 2000

PocketRadiologist™
Cardiac
Top 100 Diagnoses

HYPERTENSION

Left Ventricular Hypertrophy

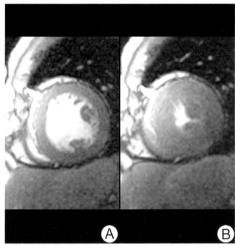

Left ventricular hypertrophy (LVH). (A) Diastolic and (B) Systolic short-axis FIESTA images demonstrate left ventricular enlargement with LV thickening and near complete obliteration of LV cavity on systolic image.

Key Facts
- Synonym(s): LVH
- Definition: Increase in left ventricular mass
- Classic imaging appearance
  - Equally distributed increase in ventricular wall thickness with normal ventricular chamber dimensions
  - Left ventricle (LV) thickening measured at end-diastole
  - LV thickness exceeding 1.1 cm indicates hypertrophy
- Left ventricular hypertrophy in patients with systemic hypertension is a significant risk factor for future morbid events

Imaging Findings
General Features
- Best imaging clue
  - End diastolic wall thickness exceeding 1.1 cm
MR Findings
- Cine-gradient echo or steady state free precession imaging
- MRI is the method of choice or precisely quantifying LV mass
- LV mass
  - Males 148 +/- 26 gm (76 +/- 13 gm/m^2)
  - Females 108 +/- 21 gm (66 +/- 11 gm/m^2)
- Normal end-diastolic wall thickness = 0.7 - 1.1 cm
  - Mild LVH = 1.2-1.4 cm
  - Moderate LVH = 1.5-1.9 cm
  - Severe LVH $\geq$ 2 cm
- Relative wall thickness
  - Eccentric hypertrophy < 0.30
  - Normal 0.3-0.45
  - Concentric hypertrophy > 0.45

Left Ventricular Hypertrophy

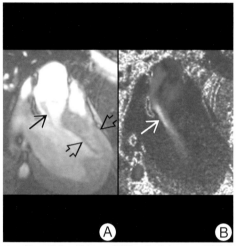

LV hypertrophy with aortic insufficiency. (A) Magnitude image and (B) phase-velocity reconstruction demonstrates regurgitant jet associated with aortic insufficiency (arrow). Note the eccentric hypertrophy of the LV with marked thickening and globular configuration (open arrows) seen in LVH associated with valvular insufficiency.

Other Modality Findings
- Echocardiography
  - o Mainstay for evaluating left ventricular function
  - o Same findings as described for MRI

Differential Diagnosis
Hypertrophic Cardiomyopathy
- Asymmetric pattern of hypertrophy
- Absence of hypertension
- Dynamic outflow obstruction on echo/MRI
- Abnormal diastolic function
Restrictive Cardiomyopathy
- Concentric pattern of hypertrophy
- Absence of hypertension
- Right ventricular hypertrophy often present
- Abnormal diastolic function

Pathology
General
- Etiology-Pathogenesis
  - o Systemic hypertension most common cause of left ventricular hypertrophy
  - o Less common causes include valvular stenosis or regurgitation
- Epidemiology
  - o 62 million persons in the United States have systemic hypertension
  - o 40% of African-American males over age 50 have systemic hypertension
Gross Pathologic, Surgical Features
- Characterization of hypertrophy
  - o Concentric hypertrophy

Left Ventricular Hypertrophy

- Uniform increase in ventricular wall thickness
- Normal ventricular chamber dimension
- Increased ventricular mass
  o Concentric remodeling
    - Normal chamber dimensions
    - Increase in relative wall thickness
    - Normal ventricular mass
    - Patients with hypertension, reduced cardiac output, and high peripheral vascular resistance
  o Eccentric hypertrophy
    - Increased ventricular dimensions
    - Normal wall thickness
    - Low or normal relative wall thickness
    - Increased ventricular mass
    - Seen in patients with valvular regurgitation
  o Asymmetric hypertrophy
    - Nonuniform increase in wall thickness
    - Associated with hypertrophic cardiomyopathy

Clinical Issues

Presentation
- Hypertension (systolic BP > 140 mmHg, diastolic BP > 90 mmHg)
- Left ventricular hypertrophy on EKG

Treatment
- Treat underlying cause
- Medical therapy for hypertension
- Surgical therapy for valvular disease as indicated

Prognosis
- Good

Selected References
1. Otto CM: Cardiomyopathies, hypertensive and pulmonary heart disease. In: Textbook of Clinical Echocardiography, 2nd Ed. W.B. Saunders, Philadelphia, 183-203, 2000
2. Devereux RB et al: Left ventricular hypertrophy and hypertension. Clin Exp Hypertens 15:1025-32, 1993

Right Ventricular Hypertrophy

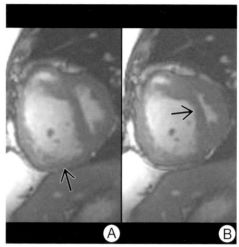

Right ventricular hypertrophy. (A) End-diastolic short-axis image shows enlargement of the right ventricle with thickening of right ventricular free wall, which exceeds 7 mm (arrow). (B) End-systolic short-axis image demonstrates "D" configuration of left ventricle and paradoxical motion of the interventricular septum (arrow).

Key Facts
- Synonym(s): RVH
- Definition: Increased right ventricular myocardial mass and wall thickness
- Other key facts
  - Normal right ventricle (RV) free wall mass = 26 +/- 5 gm/m^2
  - Normal RV free wall thickness < 6 mm

Imaging Findings
General Features
- Best imaging clue: Right ventricular free wall thickness > 7 mm as assessed on MRI, the best method for evaluating the RV
MR Findings
- Short-access cine-gradient echo imaging optimal method for assessing right ventricular mass and thickness (now SSFP: True FISP, FIESTA, Balanced FE)
- Temporal resolution should be 25-40 m sec in order to accurately assess systole and diastole time points
- Normal RV functional parameters
  - RV end-diastolic volume 138 +/- 40 ml
  - RV end-systolic volume 54 +/- 21 ml
  - RV free wall mass 46 +/- 11 gm (26 +/- 5 gm/m^2)
  - RV ejection fraction (%) = 61 +/- 7
  - RV stroke volume = 84 +/- 24 ml (46 +/- 8 ml/m^2)

Differential Diagnosis
RVH Due to Pulmonary Hypertension
- RV mass exceeds 60 gm
- Pulmonary artery (PA) pressure estimated as $(P_{right\ atrium}) + 4\ V^2$
  - V is peak velocity of regurgitant tricuspid valve jet

Right Ventricular Hypertrophy

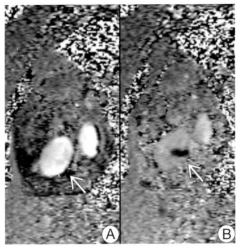

Estimation of right ventricle (RV) Pressure from velocity of tricuspid regurgitant jet. (A) Diastolic and (B) systolic phase-velocity images in short-axis at atrial ventricular level. (A) Diastolic image shows normal filling of RV (arrow). (B) Systolic image demonstrates regurgitant jet (arrow) associated with tricuspid regurgitation.

- o Right atrial pressure ($P_{right atrium}$) estimated by size of inferior vena cava IVC
  - ▪ Small   (< 1.5 cm) 0-5 mmHg
  - ▪ Normal (1.5-2.5 cm) 5-15 mmHg
  - ▪ Dilated (> 2.5 cm) 15-20 mmHg
  - ▪ Dilated, enlarged hepatic veins > 20 mmHg

Congenital Heart Disease
- Right ventricular hypertrophy a common manifestation of congenital heart disease
- Tetralogy of Fallot
- Transposition of great vessels

Pathology
General
- Etiology-Pathogenesis: RVH occurs as a result of pulmonary hypertension
  - o Congenital heart disease
  - o Primary pulmonary hypertension (etiology unknown)
  - o Secondary pulmonary hypertension
    - ▪ Acquired heart disease, especially left ventricular dysfunction
    - ▪ Valvular heart disease
    - ▪ Chronic pulmonary edema (PE)
    - ▪ Pulmonary disease
    - ▪ Chronic obstructive pulmonary disease (COPD)
    - ▪ Chronic interstitial lung disease
    - ▪ Chronic bronchitis

Clinical Issues
Presentation
- Exertional dyspnea

Right Ventricular Hypertrophy

- Chest pain
- Cor pulmonale
- Cyanosis
- Right axis deviation on EKG

Treatment
- Medical treatment
  - Treat underlying cause of secondary pulmonary hypertension
  - Pulmonary vasodilators
- Surgical treatment
  - Valve replacement
  - IVC filter for recurrent pulmonary emboli
  - Transplantation

Selected References
1. Lorenz CH: Right ventricular anatomy and function in health and disease. In: Cardiovascular Magnetic Resonance, Manning WJ, Pannell DJ, Churchill-Livingstone, Philadelphia. 283-92, 2002
2. Otto CM: Echocardiographic evaluation of left and right ventricular systolic function. In: Textbook of Clinical Echocardiography, 2nd Ed. W.B. Saunders, Philadelphia. 120-3, 2000

Pulmonary Arterial Hypertension

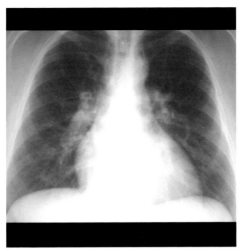

Chest x-ray demonstrates bilateral central pulmonary artery enlargement with abrupt tapering of the distal pulmonary vessels.

Key Facts
- Mean pulmonary artery hypotension (PAH) pressure > 25 mmHg at rest or > 30 mmHg during exercise
- Increased pulmonary vascular resistance; decreased cross-sectional area of capillary bed
- May be primary PAH (pPAH) = plexogenic pulmonary arteriopathy – no underlying cause can be identified
- Secondary PAH (sPAH) is caused by underlying disease (see below)
- Primary pulmonary hypertension is present if all types of secondary pulmonary hypertension have been excluded
- Classic appearance: Enlarged central pulmonary arteries, pruning of pulmonary vessels
- Right chambers enlarged if cor pulmonale develops
- Must be differentiated from pulmonary venous hypertension (PVH)
  - Redistribution of pulmonary vasculature
  - Pulmonary arteries not enlarged, unless secondary PAH develops
  - Secondary to left ventricle (LV) failure or obstructive disorders

Imaging Findings
General Features
- Large main pulmonary artery (PA), pruning of pulmonary arteries
Chest Radiography Findings
- Convex pulmonary trunk segment
- Large central pulmonary arteries (L PA > 17 mm) with rapid tapering of peripheral vessels
- Normal-sized heart or right ventricle (RV) enlargement (cor pulmonale)
Echocardiography Findings
- Signs of cor pulmonale
  - Increased thickness of RV +/- RV dilation
  - Systolic paradoxical bulging of the septum into LV ("D" sign)
  - Tricuspid regurgitation (90% of patients)

Pulmonary Arterial Hypertension

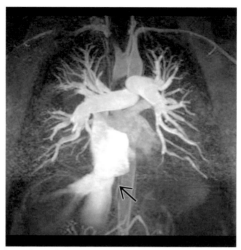

Contrast-enhanced MRA demonstrates marked pulmonary enlargement with "pruning" of the distal pulmonary vessels. Also note marked right atrial and inferior vena cava (IVC) enlargement representing elevated systemic venous pressure (arrow).

- Modified Bernoulli equation used to determine PA pressure

CT Findings
- Large central PA with disproportional small peripheral arteries
- PA wall calcification is pathognomonic
- May aid in detecting underlying cause (e.g., pulmonary fibrosis, emphysema, pulmonary embolism (PE))

MR Findings
- MRA: Proximal PA size > 28 mm, MRA may detect pulmonary embolism
- MR Phase mapping useful in estimating PA pressure

Angiography Findings
- Right heart catheterization is gold standard for measuring PA pressure
- Normal wedge pressure in pPAH
- Pulmonary angiography bears increased risk in PAH
- May show tricuspid and pulmonic regurgitation

Differential Diagnosis

Congenital Disorders
- Tetralogy variant: Markedly enlarged PAs, absence of pulmonary valve
- Pulmonary stenosis: Jet causes isolated left PA enlargement

Others
- Hilar adenopathy may mimic PAH on chest radiograph
- Partial absence of pericardium may cause convexity of left cardiac contour
  - Usually lower than main PA segment

Pathology

General
- Etiology-Pathogenesis
  - sPAH caused by
    - Pulmonary venous hypertension

- Parenchymal lung disease: Chronic obstructive pulmonary disease (COPD), emphysema, bronchiectasis, cystic fibrosis, pulmonary fibrosis, HIV infection, etc.
- Vascular obstruction: Chronic pulmonary edema (PE), venoocclusive disease, arteritis, lupus, scleroderma
- Congenital L to R shunts: Atrial septal defect (ASD), ventricular septal defect (VSD), endocardial cushion defect, etc.
- Alveolar hypoventilation: Chronic high altitudes, sleep apnea, neuromuscular disease, obesity, fibrothorax, kyphoscoliosis, etc.
  - Primary PAH unknown etiology
    - Familial occurrence suggests genetic abnormality but gene not yet identified
    - Autosomal dominant, female:male = 2:1
    - Appetite suppressants increase risk
- Epidemiology
  - Incidence of pPAH: 1-2 per million per year
  - Incidence in appetite suppressant users: 25-50 per million per year
  - Prevalence: 1300 per million

Microscopic Grading
- Grade I: Media hypertrophy of arteries + arterioles
- Grade II: Muscular hypertrophy + intimal proliferation arterioles
- Grade III: Additional subendothelial fibrosis
- Grade IV: Vessel occlusion plus small artery dilatation
- Grade V: Plexiform endothelial proliferation, tortuous channels, intra-alveolar macrophages
- Grade VI: Necrotizing arteritis with thrombosis

Clinical Issues
Presentation
- Gradual onset of dyspnea on exertion and shortness of breath (SOB)
- Usually delayed presentation 2 years after symptom onset
- Chest pain, syncope, fatigue, peripheral edema
- Ortner's syndrome: Hoarseness from compressed left recurrent laryngeal nerve by enlarged PA

Natural History
- pPAH is uniformly lethal

Treatment
- No cure for pPAH
- Medical therapy: Calcium channel blockers, epoprostenol (prostacyclin), anticoagulants, oxygen rarely of benefit
  - Only 30% respond to medical therapy
- Surgical therapy: Lung transplant, blade-balloon septostomy in severe right heart failure

Prognosis
- Median survival from diagnosis in pPAH 2.5 (US) - 3.4 years (UK)
- 95% 5 year survival for "responders" to calcium channel blockers
- Potentially lethal rebound after termination of calcium channel blockers

Selected References
1. Krüger S et al: Diagnosis of pulmonary arterial hypertension and pulmonary embolism with magnetic resonance angiograph. Chest 120 (J):1556-61, 2001
2. Webb WR et al: Pulmonary Hypertension and Pulmonary Vascular Disease. In Webb WR et al. High-Resolution CT of the Lung. 3rd ed. Lippincott Williams & Wilkins, Philadelphia, 547-67, 2001
3. Gaine SP et al: Primary pulmonary hypertension. The Lancet, 352:719-25, 1998

Branch Pulmonary Stenosis

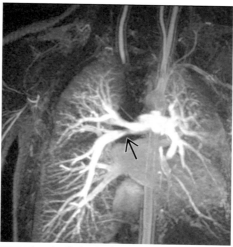

Branch pulmonary stenosis. Contrast-enhanced MRA demonstrates focal stenosis of right interlobar lobe pulmonary artery (arrow). Velocity measurements distal to stenosis indicated elevated peak systolic velocities with an estimated pressure gradient of 40 mmHg. Patient has history of arterioventricular (AV) canal repair.

Key Facts
- Definition: Stenosis of pulmonary artery and/or branches
- Classic imaging appearance
  - Focal or long-segment stenosis of pulmonary artery
  - Evidence for collateral aortopulmonary circulation to lung in chronic pulmonary artery stenosis
- Other key facts
  - Common anatomic component of complex cyanotic congenital heart disease
  - Common long-term complication of congenital heart disease

Imaging Findings
General Features
- Best imaging clue: Stenosis of pulmonary artery
CT Findings
- NECT: May see calcification in setting of fibrosing mediastinitis
- CTA: Similar to MRA
MR Findings
- T1WI: Useful for evaluating soft tissue anatomy of mediastinum or lesions surrounding stenosed pulmonary arteries
- T2WI: Useful for characterizing lesions creating extrinsic compression of pulmonary arteries
- MRA
  - Focal or diffuse stenosis involving pulmonary artery
  - Focal or diffuse stenosis of pulmonary veins
  - Evidence for aortopulmonary collateral circulation in chronic pulmonary artery stenosis
  - Contrast-enhanced 3D MRA technique shown to be as accurate as conventional arteriography for detecting pulmonary stenoses and aorto-pulmonary collaterals

Branch Pulmonary Stenosis

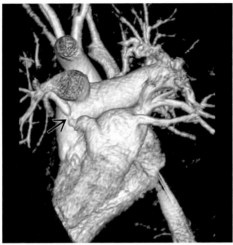

Pulmonary vein stenosis in patient following reanastomosis of anomalous left upper lobe vein to left atrium. Posterior view from volume-rendered MRA demonstrates focal stenosis at surgical anastomosis between anomalous left upper lobe pulmonary vein and left atrium (arrow). Note normal contralateral pulmonary veins.

- o Phase-contrast velocity measurement important to characterize the hemodynamic significance of pulmonary stenosis
  - ▪ Peak systolic velocities exceeding 1.5 mm/sec imply hemodynamically significant stenosis
  - ▪ Cine-gradient-echo imaging may be helpful for characterizing associated congenital heart abnormalities
- o Noncontrast MRA of limited value

Other Modality Findings
- Echocardiography has limited usefulness due to limited acoustic window for evaluating branch pulmonary stenosis

Imaging Recommendations
- Routine spin echo and cine MRI followed by contrast-enhanced 3D MRA

Differential Diagnosis
Isolated Pulmonary Stenosis
- Unusual cause of pulmonary stenosis

Pulmonary Stenosis Associated with Congenital Heart Disease
- Tetralogy of Fallot
- Pulmonary atresia
- Post-Fontan pulmonary palliation

Adult-Acquired Pulmonary Stenosis
- Chronic pulmonary embolism
- Vasculitis
  - o Takayasu's arteritis
    - ▪ Young to middle-aged women
    - ▪ Pulmonary arteries affected in > 50% of cases
    - ▪ Usually bilateral and multifocal
    - ▪ Predilection for upper lobe branches

Branch Pulmonary Stenosis

- o Connective tissue disorders
  - Scleroderma
  - Rheumatoid arthritis
  - Systemic lupus erythematosus
- o Behcet disease
- o Wegener's granulomatosis
- o Allergic angiitis and granulomatosis

Pulmonary Vein Stenosis
- Patients post-radiofrequency ablation of ectopic atrial foci
- Patients following re-anastomosis of anomalous pulmonary vein

Pathology

General
- Etiology-Pathogenesis
  - o Most common cause is abnormal pulmonary circulation in congenital heart disease
  - o Stenosis may be acquired, especially in presence of pulmonary revascularization procedures (Fontan, Blalock-Taussig shunt)

Gross Pathologic, Surgical Features
- Narrowing of pulmonary artery or branches
- Thickening of pulmonary arterial wall
- Aortopulmonary collateral circulation through bronchial arteries

Microscopic Features
- Inflammation of vessel wall in setting of vasculitis

Clinical Issues

Presentation
- Cyanotic congenital heart disease
- Features of systemic vasculitis
- Presentation of pulmonary vein stenosis related to venous hypertension
  - o Pleural effusions
  - o Pulmonary edema, unilateral or asymmetric

Treatment
- Percutaneous balloon angioplasty
- Surgical revascularization for proximal pulmonary artery stenosis/atresia associated with congenital heart disease

Prognosis
- Branch pulmonary stenosis is a serious and long-term complication of congenital heart disease
- Prognosis is poor

Selected References
1. Geva T et al: Gadolinium-enhanced 3-dimensional magnetic resonance angiography of pulmonary blood supply in patients with complex pulmonary stenosis or atresia: Comparison with X-ray angiography. Circulation 106:473-8, 2002
2. Bacha EA et al: Comprehensive management of branch pulmonary artery stenosis. J Interv Cardiol 14(3):367-75, 2001

PocketRadiologist™
Cardiac
Top 100 Diagnoses

VASCULAR DISEASE

Carotid Stenosis

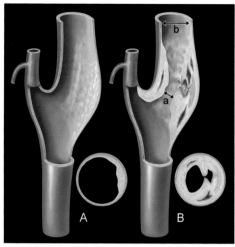

Graphic depiction of mild and severe carotid atherosclerosis (ASVD). (A) Earliest signs of ASVD are "fatty streaks" and slight intimal thickening. (B) Severe stenosis with intraplaque hemorrhage, ulceration and platelet emboli are shown. NASCET calculation % stenosis=(b-a)/b x 100.

Key Facts
- Stroke is second most common worldwide cause of death
- Most cerebral infarcts occur in carotid vascular territory
- Carotid stenosis =/> 70% associated with significant stroke risk, benefit from endarterectomy

Imaging Findings
General Features
- Smooth or irregular narrowing of internal carotid artery (ICA) origin

CT Findings
- +/- Ca++ in vessel wall
- Large plaques may show low density foci

MR Findings
- MRA provides multidirectional imaging (vs. conventional DSA)
- "Flow gap" (loss of signal) in cases of high-grade stenosis
- Signal loss can occur if artery narrowed (> 95%) but not occluded
- Brain T2WI, FLAIR may show "rosary-like" lesions in centrum semiovale ipsilateral to stenosis (hemodynamic failure)
- Contrast-enhanced MRA best for demonstrating origins carotid arteries
  - Tandem lesions in 10-20%
  - CEMRA also improves delineation of complex morphology

Other Modality Findings
- CTA
  - Demonstrates lumen
  - Wall Ca++ identified
  - Patchy/homogeneous low density in wall often seen with large necrotic/lipid plaque
  - Poor correlation with ulceration
- DSA

Carotid Stenosis

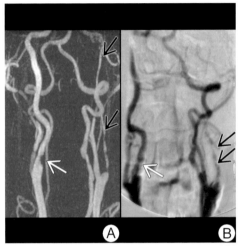

Carotid stenosis with "string sign". (A) Time-resolved CE-MRA and (B) x-ray DSA. (A) The left ICA shows a severe stenosis with delayed filling of the distal ICA (black arrows) Note stenosis of the right ICA (white arrow). (B) DSA shows poor filling in distal left ICA (black arrows) and the right ICA stenosis (white arrow).

- Current standard of reference (N.B.: Enhanced CTA, MRA adequate for evaluation of carotid stenosis)
- Role of DSA
  - Evaluate great vessel origins
  - Calculate % carotid stenosis
  - At least 4 projections (AP, lateral, both obliques) recommended
  - Maximum narrowing used
- Identify "tandem" distal ICA stenosis (2% of cases)
- Depict presence of collateral flow (lower risk of stroke, TIA)
- Detect other lesions (e.g., aneurysm)
- Calculating carotid stenosis
  - Methods vary (NASCET vs. European trials)
- Irregular plaque surface = increased stroke risk on medical Rx at all degrees of stenosis
- Pseudoocclusion
  - Very high-grade stenosis
  - Slow antegrade "trickle" of contrast may be shown only on late phase of angiogram
  - Important because endarterectomy an option if ICA still patent
  - High stroke risk

Imaging Recommendations
- Ultrasound as screening tool
- CTA/MRA
- DSA if CTA/MRA show "occlusion"

Differential Diagnosis

Extrinsic Compressive Lesion (Rare)
- Carotid space neoplasm

Carotid Stenosis

Dissection
- Typically spares bulb, ICA origin (atherosclerosis involves both)
- No Ca++
- "Flame shaped" ICA

Pathology
General
- General path comments
  - Significant ICA narrowing identified in 20%-30% of carotid territory strokes (vs. 5-10% of general population)
- Etiology-Pathogenesis-Pathophysiology
  - Risk of stroke increases with stenosis severity
    - Hypoperfusion
    - Artery-to-artery emboli
  - Stenosis is not sole factor (plaque morphology also correlated)

Gross Pathologic, Surgical Features
- See "Penetrating Ulcer"

Microscopic Features
- See "Penetrating Ulcer"

Clinical Issues
Presentation
- TIA
- Stroke (can be silent)

Natural History
- Progressive

Treatment & Prognosis
- NASCET
  - Symptomatic stenosis = 70% benefits from endarterectomy
  - Symptomatic moderate stenosis (50-69%) also benefits from endarterectomy, but less
- ACAS
  - Asymptomatic patients benefit even with stenosis of 60%

Selected References
1. Randoux B et al: Carotid artery stenosis: Prospective comparison of CT, gadolinium-enhanced MR, and conventional angiography. Radiology 220:179-85, 2001
2. Rothwell PM et al: Interrelation between plaque surface morphology and degree of stenosis on carotid angiograms and the risk of ischemic stroke in patients with symptomatic carotid stenosis. Stroke 31:615-21, 2000
3. Rothwell PM et al: Critical appraisal of the design and reporting of studies of imaging and measurement of carotid stenosis. Stroke 31:1444-50, 2000

Subclavian Steal Syndrome (SSS)

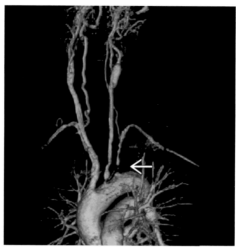

Volume rendered display of aortic arch shows high-grade stenosis (arrow) of left subclavian artery. Left common carotid artery is stenotic as well.

Key Facts
- Collateral blood flow to the arm from reversed flow in vertebral artery (VA) secondary to occlusion or stenosis of subclavian artery (SCA) proximal to VA orifice
- Steal of blood through circle of Willis causes transient vertebrobasilar cerebral symptoms upon exercising the ipsilateral upper extremity
- Arteriogram shows cutoff of SCA and absence of VA on early images; later phase shows reversed flow of contrast through VA filling the distal SCA

Imaging Findings
General Features
- Delayed contrast imaging is essential
- Steal may be only apparent if upper extremity is exercised or reactive hyperemia induced (blood pressure cuff inflated above systolic arterial pressure for > 5 min)

Chest Radiography Finding
- No specific signs

Angiography Findings
- SCA stenosis or occlusion proximal to VA
- Later phase demonstrates retrograde filling of VA and distal SCA
- Territory from which steal occurs: Vertebro-vertebral, carotid basilar, external carotid-vertebral and carotid subclavian (with brachiocephalic occlusion)
- Pitfall: "False steal" may occur in selective VA injection - high injection pressure transiently reverses flow in contralateral VA

Duplex Ultrasound Findings
- Transient decrease in ipsilateral vertebral artery midsystolic velocity is earliest sign
- Reversed flow in ipsilateral VA
- Arm exercise exaggerates waveform changes

Subclavian Steal Syndrome (SSS)

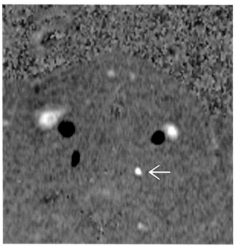

Phase-contrast MRI demonstrates retrograde flow of blood in the vertebral artery, due to subclavian steal syndrome. Left vertebral artery (arrow) shows bright signal, in opposite direction to right.

- Increased blood flow in the contralateral VA (not precisely defined, but peak systolic velocity > 60 cm/sec suggests abnormality)
- Parvus tardus waveform in distal subclavian and brachial artery

MR Findings
- Flow reversal will be inapparent on 2D time of flight MR images but will be readily apparent on phase contrast images
- Gd-enhanced MRA sensitive for depicting SCA stenosis

CT Findings
- Noncontrast CT may detect calcification of SCA, CTA can depict subclavian stenosis
- Contrast enhanced CT may mask calcification
- Absence of calcification does not exclude SSS; presence of calcification does not confirm SSS

Differential Diagnosis

Right Common Carotid Steal
- Associated with high-grade innominate artery stenosis or occlusion (right side only)
- Analogous to subclavian steal, but blood is "stolen" from the right common carotid artery (RCCA), as well as the right VA

Other Causes of Vertebrobasilar Symptoms
- Multiple sclerosis; thromboembolism; cerebellar neoplasm; cerebellar degeneration

Other Causes of Luminal Narrowing
- Tumor encasement, Trauma

Pathology

General
- General path comments
  - Left:Right = 3-4:1

Subclavian Steal Syndrome (SSS)

- o Male:Female = 3:1
- o Average age ~ 60 years
- o 81% have associated cervical artery lesions
- Causes
  - o Congenital
    - ▪ Interruption/hypoplasia of aortic arch, preductal coarctation, coarctation with distal anomalous right subclavian artery, etc.
  - o Acquired
    - ▪ Atherosclerosis (94%)
    - ▪ Arteritis: Takayasu's arteritis, giant cell arteritis
    - ▪ Previous invasive procedure or surgery
    - ▪ Blalock-Taussig shunt with ligation of SCA
    - ▪ Trauma/dissection/tumor compression
- Pathophysiology
  - o SCA stenosis causes decreased pressure in distal upper extremity arteries
  - o Collateral arterial flow through reversal of vertebral artery blood flow
  - o Neurological symptoms occur when blood flow requirement to upper extremity (UE) increases secondary to increased shunting away from circle of Willis
- Epidemiology
  - o 1.3% of patients referred for carotid/VA Doppler US; of those 5% have neurological symptoms

SSS Staging
- Stage I: Reduced antegrade flow (implies SCA stenosis)
- Stage II: "Intermittent steal" reversed flow only during reactive hyperemia testing of arm (implies SCA stenosis)
- Stage III: "Persistent steal" permanent reversed flow (implies SCA occlusion)

Clinical Issues

Presentation
- Frequently asymptomatic
- Decreased blood pressure in affected UE
- Weak or absent pulse, pain, paresthesia, weakness, coolness, numbness in arm
- Vertebrobasilar symptoms
  - o Syncopes when exercising arm
  - o Headache, nausea, vertigo, ataxia, diplopia, homonymous hemianopia, perioral paresthesia, dysphagia, dysarthria

Treatment
- Balloon angioplasty +/- stent
- Surgical bypass: common carotid to SCA or innominate to SCA

Prognosis
- Good results after bypass surgery or percutaneous transluminal angioplasty (PTA) (patency rate 94% and 86%)
- Underlying disease may be progressive

Selected References
1. Kliewer, MA et al: Vertebral artery Doppler waveform changes indicating subclavian steal physiology. AJR 174:815-19, 2000
2. Dähnert WF: Radiology Review Manual 4th Ed., Lippincott Williams & Wilkins, Philadelphia, 537-8, 1999

Cervical Artery Dissection

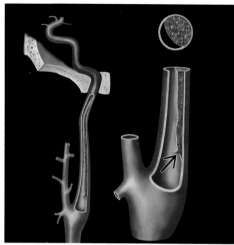

Graphic depicts subintimal dissection of the cervical ICA. Note proximal intimal tear (arrow), eccentric ICA narrowing. The bulb is spared and the dissection ends at the skull base.

Key Facts
- Internal carotid artery is most frequent site of craniocervical artery dissection
- Dissection causes 10-25% of ischemic strokes in young adults
- Consider in young/middle-aged patient with headache, TIA
- Stroke from vertebral artery dissection often preceded by neck pain, vertigo and unilateral facial paresthesia

Imaging Findings
General Features
- Tubular narrowing that spares bulb, stops at skull base
- Secondary emboli, stroke common

CT Findings
- Noncontrast CT may be negative
- Contrast-enhanced CT may show true, false lumen separated by linear lucency

MR Findings
- Crescentic intramural hematoma
  - Acute clot iso-, subacute hyperintense on T1WI, T2WI
- Eccentrically narrowed residual lumen
  - May have absent/diminished "flow void"
  - Slow flow may cause intravascular signal

Angiography (DSA/CTA/MRA) Findings
- String sign: Smooth or irregular tapered narrowing extending to skull base
- Internal carotid artery (ICA) dissection usually spares bulb
- Intimal flap may be visible and create double-barrel lumen
- May have extraluminal pouch (dissecting aneurysm)
  - May occlude true lumen

Cervical Artery Dissection

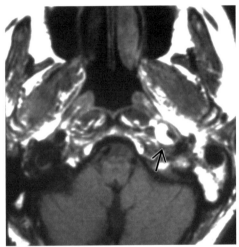

Dissection on T1WI. Note the high signal intensity associated with subacute thrombus in the false channel of the carotid dissection (arrow).

<u>Imaging Recommendations</u>
- MR (fat-suppressed T1WI helpful for subacute clot), MRA
- DSA if MR/MRA negative

Differential Diagnosis
<u>Fibromuscular Dysplasia (FMD)</u>
- "String of beads" appearance > long tubular narrowing
<u>Thrombosis</u>
- Often involves bulb
- IA contrast may delineate intraluminal clot, meniscus
<u>Atherosclerosis</u>
- Involves bulb
- Irregular > smooth tapered narrowing
- Ca++ often present
<u>Vasospasm</u>
- (Migraine, catheter-induced, etc.)

Pathology
<u>General</u>
- General path comments
  - Can occur between or within any layers
    - Subintimal > subadventitial
  - Mid-cervical ICA > vertebral artery (VA) (skull base/C1, C1-2 most common)
    - 15% multiple vessels
  - Rare: Intracranial dissection
- Etiology-Pathogenesis
  - Congenital/acquired defect in internal elastic lamina
  - Trauma
    - Penetrating or blunt, stretching/torsion (including chiropractic manipulation which affects VA > ICA)

- Minor neck torsion, trivial trauma in 25% (intense physical activity, coughing, sneezing)
  - o "Spontaneous"
    - Underlying vasculopathy common (e.g., FMD, Marfan, Ehlers-Danlos)
    - Increased plasma homocysteine levels
    - Familial ICA dissection may occur
    - Hypertension in 1/3 of all patients
- Epidemiology
  - o Annual incidence = 3.5 per 100,000

Gross Pathologic, Surgical Features
- Long segment narrowing with intramural clot

Clinical Issues

Presentation
- 70% of patients between 35-50 years with equal male:female ratio
- Headache, neck/facial pain or numbness
  - o 60-90% of patients with cervical ICA dissection
  - o Onset a few hours up to 3-4 weeks
- Horner's in 1/3
- Uncommon: Cranial nerve palsy (CN XII > IX, X, XI)
- Ischemic symptoms may occur as complication
- Vertebral dissection also: Dizziness/vertigo, nausea, diplopia, extremity weakness/numbness/dysarthria

Natural History
- Usually resolves spontaneously (6-8 weeks)

Treatment & Prognosis
- Treatment: Antithrombotics
- Prognosis
  - o No residual or mild neurologic deficit in 70%
  - o Disabling in 25%
  - o Fatal in 5%

Selected References
1. Bin Saeed A et al: Vertebral artery dissection: Warning symptoms, clinical features and prognosis in 26 Patients. Can J Neurol Sci 27:292-6, 2000
2. Lee WW et al: Bilateral internal carotid artery dissection due to trivial trauma. J Emerg Med 19:35-41, 2000
3. Oelerich M et al: Craniocervical artery dissection: MR imaging and MR angiographic findings. Eur Radiol 9:1385-91, 1999

Thoracic Outlet Syndrome (TOS)

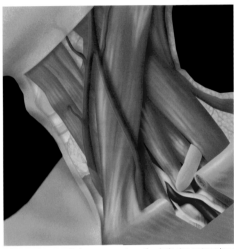

Thoracic outlet syndrome. Note compression of subclavian artery by cervical rib.

Key Facts
- Upper extremity (UE) impingement syndrome involving the brachial plexus, subclavian artery, vein or lymphatics
- 95% neurological impairment, 5% vascular compression
- May lead to subclavian vein (SCV) thrombosis (3.5% of cases R:L = 3:2)
- Subclavian artery intimal damage may lead to premature atherosclerosis, stenosis or occlusion, post stenotic ectasia or aneurysm and distal embolization

Imaging Findings
General Features
- Provocative maneuvers may be needed during diagnostic tests to induce compression of subclavian artery/vein
  - Adson's maneuver: Extension of neck and rotation of head towards affected side +/- deep inspiration/downward traction on arm
  - Allen test: Arm is raised and rotated while the head is turned to the opposite side
- Nerve conduction velocity testing may be helpful

Chest Radiography Findings
- Usually no specific findings
- Presence of cervical rib, nonanatomically healed rib, clavicle or scapular fractures, exuberant callus, etc.

CT Findings
- Detection of neoplasms or osseous anomalies: Congenital variants, callous formation, exostosis, degenerative spine changes
- CTA may demonstrate stenosis/distal aneurysm/thrombus
- Scanning before and after postural maneuvers shows significant change of costosubclavian distance (subclavius muscle to 1st rib)
- Frontal and superior volume rendered CTA images allow assessment of course changes of subclavian artery in respect to bony landmarks

Thoracic Outlet Syndrome (TOS)

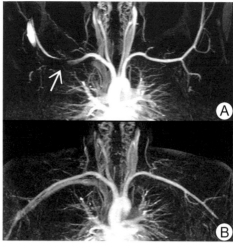

Thoracic outlet syndrome. Contrast-enhanced MRA exams obtained during abduction of the arms (A), and with arms at side (B). Note the occlusion of the right subclavian artery (arrow) during abduction. In addition, venous pooling associated with venous stasis is noted on the right.

MR Findings
- Combination of 3D time-resolved Gd-MRA and T1W spin-echo imaging used to interrogate for vascular compromise +/- provocative maneuvers
- Coronal reconstruction allows for detection of brachial plexus compression
- Minimum distance between 1st rib and clavicle in sagittal plane < 20 mm suggests TOS

Angiography Findings
- May be normal in neutral position
- Smooth extrinsic compression of artery/vein with provocative maneuver
- Distal arterial aneurysm +/- mural thrombus
- Distal UE embolization possible
- Subclavian vein thrombosis = "effort thrombosis" or "Paget von Schrötter Syndrome"

Differential Diagnosis
Neurological Disease
- Cervical radiculopathy
- Sudeck's dystrophy
- Brachial plexus injury
Neoplasm
- Spinal cord tumor
- Pancoast tumor
Vascular Disease
- Aneurysm/thromboembolism
- Vasculitis, Raynaud's disease
- Atherosclerosis

Thoracic Outlet Syndrome (TOS)

Pathology

General

- Age 10-50 years
- Female-to-male ratio 3:1; except venous subgroup 1:3
- Etiology
  - Congenital anatomical narrowing
    - Interscalene triangle: Scalenus anticus muscular hypertrophy causes compression of brachial plexus/subclavian artery
    - Cervical rib: Osseous anomaly causing compression of subclavian artery +/- lower components of brachial plexus
    - Costoclavicular syndrome: Retroclavicular compression of subclavian artery and vein by costoclavicular ligament
    - Subcoracoid tunnel: Choroid processes impinges on axillary artery and vein
- Acquired causes
  - Trauma: Rib or clavicular fractures with callous formation or non-anatomical healing; effort thrombosis (SCV)
  - Hyperabduction syndrome – prolonged hyperabduction of UE causing compression of subclavian vessels/brachial plexus by clavicle, pectoralis minor or coracoid processes
  - Neoplasm: Neck mass compressing neurovascular bundle
  - Muscular body habitus causing compression at pectoralis minor tunnel
- Pathogenesis
  - External compression of any cause in neck/shoulder region
  - SCV thrombosis may develop secondary to endothelial damage from repetitive trauma/chronic compression

Clinical Issues

Presentation

- Motor symptoms: Exercise-related muscle claudication, reduced shoulder movement, fatigability, muscle wasting
- Sensory: Pain/paresthesia
- Vasomotor symptoms: Pallor, coolness, Raynaud's phenomenon, blue fingers, absent pulse, positional arm swelling

Treatment

- Physiotherapy and nonsteroidal antiinflammatory drugs
- Surgical decompression: Scalenectomy, first rib resection

Prognosis

- Excellent

Selected References

1. Demondion X et al: Thoracic outlet: Anatomic correlation with MR imaging. AJR 175:417-22, 2002
2. Remy-Jardin M et al: Helical CT angiography of thoracic outlet syndrome: Functional Anatomy. AJR 174:1667-74, 2000
3. Valji K: Vascular and Interventional Radiology. W.B. Saunders Company, Philadelphia, 1999

Takayasu's Arteritis

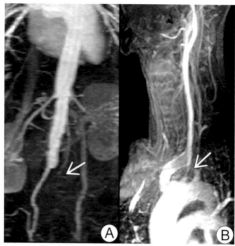

Takayasu's arteritis. (A) Contrast enhanced MRA shows infrarenal aortic narrowing with occlusion of left common iliac artery (arrow). (B) Patient also had severe stenoses of the aortic arch origin vessels, including left common carotid (arrow).

Key Facts
- Synonym: Nonspecific aortitis or aortoarteritis
- Cause
  - Unknown, but probably autoimmune
  - Primarily affects the aorta, major branches, and pulmonary arteries
  - Chronic phase results in long, smooth stenosis and occlusions of affected vessels
- Definition
  - Chronic inflammation of large elastic arterial wall

Imaging Findings
Conventional Angiography Findings
- Smooth, long stenoses of the aorta and proximal large branch vessels
- Aneurysms of proximal aorta
- Occlusions of branch vessels
- Collateral vessel formation

MRA Findings
- Diagnostic modality of choice for following response to therapy
- MRA shows features similar to conventional angiography
- MRI of vessel wall useful for following response to therapy
  - Inversion recovery T2-weighted imaging identifies inflamed vessel wall
  - T1 imaging demarcates vessel wall thickness

CTA Findings
- Findings similar to conventional angiography and MRA

Differential Diagnosis
Giant Cell Arteritis (Temporal Arteritis)
- Pathology similar to Takayasu's, with early cellular infiltration followed by vessel occlusion of medium sized vessels

Takayasu's Arteritis

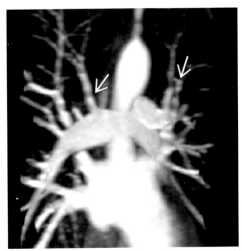

Contrast-enhanced pulmonary MRA from same patient demonstrates multiple stenoses of pulmonary arteries (arrows).

- Anatomic distribution of giant cell is different than Takayasu's
  - Involvement of intracranial vessels
  - Subclavian artery
- Predilection for elderly females rather than young
- Clinical presentation
  - Fever
  - Polymyalgia rheumatica
  - Visual changes
  - Headaches

Buerger's Disease (Thoromboangiitis Obliterans)
- Affects peripheral vessels, especially lower leg
- Originally described in younger men, but also affects woman
- Almost all patients are heavy smokers
- Vessel wall infiltration and intraluminal thrombosis
- Involves vessels distal to knee and elbow
- Abrupt occlusion of distal arteries with skip areas
- Corkscrew collaterals

Polyarteritis Nodosa (PAN)
- Necrotizing vasculitis
- Small vessel microaneurysms and intermittent occlusions
- Involvement of the kidneys, spleen, liver
- Associated with hepatitis infection

Pathology
General
- Cause unknown, but probably autoimmune
- Epidemiology
  - Strong predilection for young adult females
  - Seen most commonly in Asians, but increasing frequency in Western world

Takayasu's Arteritis

<u>Gross Pathologic, Surgical Features</u>
• Vessel occlusion
• Thickened arterial wall

<u>Microscopic Features</u>
• Acute phase
  o Media and adventitia are infiltrated with giant cells and granulomas
• Chronic phase
  o Destruction of vessel wall with adventitial fibrosis

Clinical Issues
<u>Presentation</u>
• Headaches
• Upper extremity ischemia
• Renovascular hypertension
• Intestinal ischemia
• Angina

<u>Natural History</u>
• Progressive occlusive disease
• Intermittent quiescent periods on treatment

<u>Treatment</u>
• Medical therapy aimed at reducing vessel wall inflammation
• Arterial obstructions treated when present with end-organ ischemia
• Aneurysms rarely rupture, and therefore are infrequently treated

<u>Prognosis</u>
• Patients eventually succumb to complications of chronic occlusive disease

Selected References
1.   Valji K et al: Pathogenesis of Vascular Disease in Vascular and Interventional Radiology. W.B. Saunders, Philadelphia. 47-8, 1999
2.   Hallisey MJ et al: The Abnormal Abdominal Aorta: Arteriosclerosis and Other Diseases in Abrams' Angiography. 4th ed., Baum S., Editor. Little, Brown and Company, Boston. 1054, 1997
3.   Calabrese LH et al: Systemic Vasculitis in Young J et al Peripheral Vascular Diseases. 2nd Ed., 396-401, 1996

Aortic Dissection

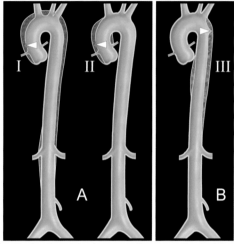

Stanford Classification Type A involves ascending aorta. Stanford Type B involves descending aorta only. DeBakey Classification Types I and II involves ascending aorta with or without descending aorta. DeBakey Type III involves descending thoracic aorta only. Intimal flap (arrow).

Key Facts
- Definition: Spontaneous longitudinal separation of aortic intima and adventitia by circulating blood
- Classic imaging appearance: Intimal flap separates true and false lumen
- Other key facts
  - Intimal flap demonstrated in 85-90%
  - False lumen generally larger and compresses true lumen
  - Majority are spontaneous
  - 2/3 dissections involve ascending aorta

Imaging Findings
Chest Radiography Findings
- Normal in 25%
- Widening superior mediastinum up to 80%
- Disparity in size between ascending and descending aorta
- Displacement of calcified mural plaque by flap > 1 cm in 7%
- Aortic silhouette enlargement on serial CXR
CT Findings
- NECT
  - Acute flap may appear hyperdense
  - IV contrast required to definitively characterize flap
  - Displacement of calcified intima
- CECT
  - 87-94% accuracy
  - "Double barrel" aorta with true and false lumen
  - Branch vessel involvement well demonstrated
  - Delayed contrast passage through false lumen
MR Findings
- T1WI

Aortic Dissection

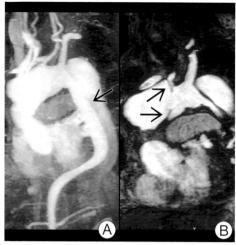

Aortic Dissection (A) MIP and (B) source image from CE-MRA shows early opacification of the true lumen. Note the MIP image in (A) obscures the dissection flap involving the ascending aorta, which is readily seen on the source image in (B) (arrows).

- Cardiac-gated black blood sequence > 95% accurate
- Contrast-enhanced MRA
  - Good for extent of dissection and involvement of branch vessels
  - 3D scan may miss ascending aortic flap due to motion
- Cine gradient echo images accurate for flap detection and valvular involvement

Echocardiography Findings
- Transthoracic echo 59-85% sensitive
- Transesophageal echo > 95% accurate
- Highly accurate for demonstrating aortic valve involvement

Angiography Findings
- Intimal flap detected in 85-90%
- Delayed filling of false lumen
- Displacement of catheter from apparent aortic wall by false lumen
- Highly accurate for entry and exit sites

Imaging Recommendations
- Primary question is defining involvement of ascending aorta
- Classically angiography was gold standard but modern cross-sectional imaging is now accepted as primary acute imaging modality

Differential Diagnosis

Hypertension
- 60-90% etiology

Collagen Disorders
- Marfan's, Ehlers-Danlos

Pregnancy
- 50% of dissections in women occur during pregnancy

Congenital
- Bicuspid aortic valve

Aortic Dissection

- Aortic coarctation
- Valvular aortic stenosis
- Turner's syndrome

Trauma
- Rare cause of dissection

Pathology
General
- General path comments
  - Transverse tear in weakened intima 95-97%, no intimal tear in 3-5%
- Etiology-Pathogenesis
  - Medial degeneration
  - Stress within aortic wall secondary to motion
  - Hydrodynamic forces accentuated by hypertension
- Epidemiology: M:F = 3:1, Peak age 60 yrs

Staging Criteria
- Stanford Classification (now preferred classification method)
  - Type A: Originates in ascending thoracic aorta (60-70%)
  - Type B: Originates distal to left subclavian artery (30-40%)
- DeBakey Classification
  - Type 1: Ascending and descending thoracic aorta (30-40%)
  - Type 2: Ascending only (10-20%)
  - Type 3: Descending only (40-50%)

Clinical Issues
Presentation
- Chest or back pain 80-90%
- Murmur in 65% secondary to aortic regurgitation
- Discrepancy between extremity pulses
- Neurologic deficits
- Silent dissections very rare

Natural History
- Complications
  - Occluded branch vessels
  - Aneurysmal enlargement of false lumen
  - Aortic valve insufficiency
  - Pericardial tamponade
  - Aortic rupture

Treatment
- Type A: Surgical placement of tubular interposition graft
- Type B: Control blood pressure, surgery if dissecting aneurysm larger than 5 cm or increasing in size by > 1.0 cm/year

Prognosis
- Without treatment
  - 24-hour mortality rate 30%, 3-month mortality rate 80%
- Long term survival in patients with operative management = 50%

Selected References
1. Kato N et al: Treatment of chronic aortic dissection by transluminal endovascular stent-graft placement: Preliminary results. JVIR 12(7):835-40, 2001
2. Dahnert WF: Radiology Review Manual 4th Ed., Lippincott Williams & Wilkins, Philadelphia, 509-11, 1999
3. Neinaber CA et al: The diagnosis of thoracic aortic dissection by non-invasive imaging procedures. N Engl J Med 328:1-5, 140-9, 1993

Thoracic Aortic Aneurysm

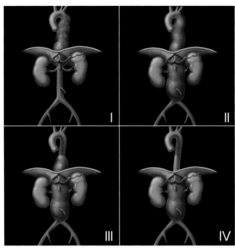

Crawford classification of TAA. (I) Descending thoracic and proximal abdominal aorta, (II) all descending and all abdominal, (III) distal descending and all abdominal aorta, (IV) abdominal aorta.

Key Facts
- Synonym(s): TAA
- Definition: Focal widening > 3cm or > 1.5x diameter of adjacent vessel
- Classic imaging appearance
  - Saccular = involvement of portion of wall
  - Fusiform = circumferential involvement
  - True aneurysm = all layers of weakened but intact walls
  - False aneurysm = focal contained perforation
- Other key facts
  - Risk of rupture increases sharply for aneurysms > 5-6 cm
  - Descending aneurysm repair indicated for > 6-7 cm
  - Surgery indicated if aneurysm grows at > 1 cm/yr

Imaging Findings
CT Findings
- NECT
  - Crescent sign = peripheral high mural attenuation indicating impending rupture due to acute intramural hematoma
  - Limited to evaluate branch vessel stenosis/occlusion
- CECT
  - Depicts luminal thrombus (80%) and branch vessel stenoses
  - Active leak depicted as extraluminal contrast
Other Modality Findings
- Plain x-ray: Mural calcification 86%
- Gd-enhanced MRA is comparable to CECT
Imaging Recommendations
- Cross-sectional imaging (MRI/MRA or CT/CTA) required to accurately characterize aneurysm

Thoracic Aortic Aneurysm

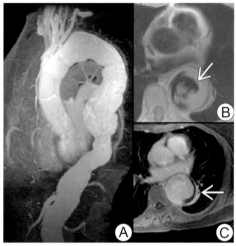

Thoracic aortic aneurysm. (A) MIP image from MRA shows descending thoracic aortic aneurysm. (B) Spin echo image shows signal in lumen of aneurysm due to slow flow (arrow). (C) Axial image shows thrombus in the lateral wall of aneurysm (arrow).

Differential Diagnosis

Atherosclerotic
- Etiology in approx 75%
- Common locations
  - Descending thoracic aorta distal to left subclavian
  - Crawford Classification System
    - Crawford 1 = all descending, some proximal abdominal
    - Crawford 2 = all descending, all abdominal
    - Crawford 3 = distal descending, some proximal abdominal
    - Crawford 4 = no descending, all abdominal

Valvular/Post-Stenotic
- Associated with aortic stenosis
- Caused by hemodynamic effect of post-stenotic jet

Infectious/Mycotic
- Bacterial: Saccular eccentric rapidly enlarging structure
- Luetic aneurysm: Ascending thoracic aneurysm that spares aortic root

Connective Tissue Disorder
- Marfan's
  - Ascending thoracic aneurysm that involves the aortic root (sino-tubular ectasia)
- Ehler-Danlos syndrome

Vasculitis
- Aneurysm formation unusual

Congenital
- Sinus of Valsalva

Pathology

General
- General path comments

- o Cystic medial degeneration is most common cause of isolated ascending thoracic aortic aneurysms
- o Increased predisposition in connective tissue and arteritis; e.g., Marfan's, Ehlers-Danlos, Takayasu's arteritis, Reiter's syndrome
- Etiology-Pathogenesis
  - o Increasing lateral hydrostatic pressure as velocity of blood flow decreases leading to compromise of mural vascular nutrition
- Epidemiology
  - o Elderly M > F

Gross Pathologic, Surgical Features
- True aneurysm all layers of aortic wall intact
- False (pseudo) aneurysm disruption of intima with contained rupture

Microscopic Features
- Diseased intima with secondary degeneration and fibrous replacement of media

Clinical Issues
Presentation
- Chest/back/shoulder pain
- Often asymptomatic, may be incidental discovery on imaging
- Symptoms of embolization
- Discovery during workup of co-existent abdominal aortic aneurysm (AAA)
- Complications
  - o Rupture
  - o Spontaneous occlusion
  - o Peripheral embolization
  - o Infection

Natural History
- Five-year survival of untreated TAA = 20%

Treatment
- Treatment recommended for diameter > 5 cm
- Bentall procedure: (Graft with prosthetic valve) for ascending aortic aneurysms that involve the sino-tubular ridge
- Inclusion graft for descending aortic aneurysms

Prognosis
- 64-94% of ruptures die outside hospital
- Surgical mortality 5-10%
- Dreaded complication of surgery is paraplegia due to spinal cord ischemia

Selected References
1. Dahnert WF et al: Radiology Review Manual, 4th Ed. Lippincott Williams & Wilkins, Philadelphia, 506-509, 1998
2. O'Hara PJ: Arterial Aneurysms in Young JR, Olin JW, Bartholomew JR. Peripheral Vascular Disease. 2nd Ed. Mosby, St Louis, MO, 349-50, 1996
3. Prince MR et al: Three-dimensional gadolinium-enhanced MR angiography of the thoracic aorta. AJR 166:1387, 1996

Mycotic Aneurysm

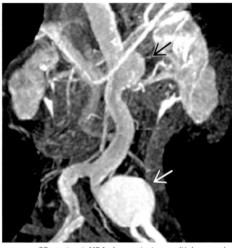

Mycotic aneurysm. 3D contrast MRA demonstrates multiple saccular aneurysms involving the aorta and left common iliac artery (arrows). This patient presented with flank pain and low-grade fever.

Key Facts
- Synonym: Infectious aneurysm (more appropriate term)
- Definition: Aneurysm arising from infection of arterial wall, usually bacterial
- Classic imaging appearance: Saccular aneurysm arising eccentrically from aortic wall
- Bacterial aortitis most commonly caused by Salmonella or Staph aureus
- Syphilitic aortitis involves the ascending aorta but spares the aortic sinus
- Ascending aorta most common location

Imaging Findings
General Features
- Best imaging clue: Rapidly growing saccular aneurysm arising eccentrically from aortic wall
CT Findings
- NECT
  - Bacterial aortitis is rarely calcified
  - Syphilitic aortitis shows curvilinear calcifications
- CECT: One or more saccular aneurysms arising form aortic wall
MR Findings
- T1WI
  - Periaortic low-signal intensity in absence of Gd
  - Aortic and periaortic enhancement following Gd, especially evident on fat-suppressed images
- T2WI: Periaortic high-signal intensity on fat-suppressed T2WI
- Contrast enhanced MRA
  - One or more saccular aneurysms arising from aortic wall
  - Effacement of wall with possible leakage at rupture site
  - It is important to review MRA as well as delayed source images to identify areas of enhancement

Mycotic Aneurysm

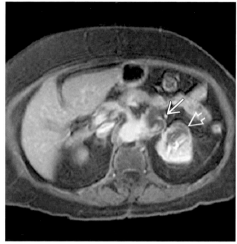

Delayed fat-suppressed T1 weighted gradient echo image in same patient as prior figure. Image demonstrates saccular aortic aneurysm (arrow) with associated renal abscess (open arrow).

<u>Imaging Recommendations</u>
- T1WI and T2WI MRI followed by contrast-enhanced MRA

Differential Diagnosis
<u>Atherosclerotic Aneurysm</u>
- Slow growing
- More often fusiform
- Often calcified
<u>Inflammatory Aneurysm</u>
- Distal aorta and iliac involvement
- Fusiform aneurysm
- Retro-peritoneal fibrosis

Pathology
<u>General</u>
- Normal aorta is resistant to infection
- Generally believed that mycotic aneurysm most often forms after diseased aorta is infected
- Etiology-Pathogenesis
  - ○ Routes of infection
    - Most often caused by seeding of an existing lesion (atheroma or aneurysm) via the vasa vasorum
    - Direct extension from infection in vessel wall, i.e., bacterial endocarditis
    - Invasion of aortic wall by extravascular contiguous infection
    - Lymphatic spread
- Epidemiology
  - ○ Increased risk in
    - IV drug abusers

Mycotic Aneurysm

- Patients with history of bacterial endocarditis
- Immunocompromised patients
- Patients with vascular prostheses (valves, grafts)

Gross Pathologic, Surgical Features
- Bacterial aneurysm
  o Non-calcified, saccular aneurysm
  o Thinning of the aortic wall with periaortic inflammatory changes
- Syphilitic aneurysm
  o Calcified lesion
  o "Tree bark" appearance when atheroma develops in infected areas

Microscopic Features
- Loss of intima and destruction of internal elastic lamina
- Media shows varying degrees of destruction
- Bacteria present on histology

Staging Criteria
- Classification system
  o Primary mycotic aneurysm arise from a distant, unknown, or remote source of infection
  o Secondary mycotic aneurysm arise from specific source of infection
    - Bacterial endocarditis (intravascular spread)
    - Tuberculosis (contiguous spread)

Clinical Issues

Presentation
- Symptoms vary greatly
- Nonspecific findings
- Low-grade fever
- Localized pain
- Positive blood cultures

Natural History
- Nearly always fatal if untreated

Treatment
- Surgical resection/grafting following antibiotic therapy

Prognosis
- Acute rupture/hemorrhage seen in 75%
- Mortality rate estimated at 67%

Selected References
1. Gonda RL et al: Mycotic aneurysm of the aorta: Radiologic features. Radiology 168:343-6, 1988
2. Vogelzang RL et al: Infected aortic aneurysm: CT appearance. JCAT 12(1):109-12, 1988
3. Lande A et al: Aortitis: Pathologic, clinical, and radiographic review. Radiol Clin North Am 14:219-40, 1976

Traumatic Aortic Laceration

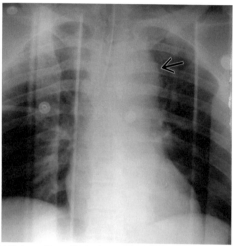

Traumatic aortic laceration. AP chest x-ray demonstrates widening of the superior mediastinum, rightward tracheal deviation and indistinct aortic knob (arrow). Patient involved in high-speed motor vehicle accident. (Courtesy of Don Yandow MD)

Key Facts
- Synonyms: Aortic pseudoaneurysm, aortic rupture, traumatic aortic aneurysm, aortic transection
- Definition: Aortic laceration or rupture secondary to sudden horizontal (MVA) or vertical (fall from great height) deceleration injury of the thorax
- Classic imaging appearance
  - Mediastinal widening
  - Localized saccular outpouching of aorta
- Location
  - 88% aortic isthmus
  - 4.5% aortic arch with avulsion of brachiocephalic trunk
  - 2% descending thoracic aorta
  - 1% ascending aorta immediately above aortic valve

Imaging Findings
Chest Radiography Findings
- Mediastinal widening > 8 cm (75%)
- Indistinct aortic outline (75% at arch, 12% at descending)
- Esophageal/nasogastric tube deviation to right (67%)
- Tracheal displacement to right (61%)
- Inferior displacement of left mainstem bronchus (53%)
- Apical pleural cap (37%)
- First or second rib fracture (17%)
CT Findings
- NECT
  - 55% sensitive, 65% specific
  - Obliteration of aortic-fat interface with increased attenuation suggesting mediastinal hemorrhage
- CECT
  - Negative CT has nearly 100% negative predictive value

Traumatic Aortic Laceration

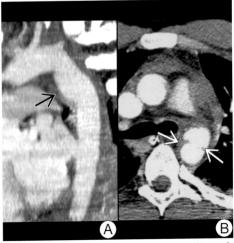

Traumatic aortic laceration. (A) Reformated image and (B) axial image from contrast-enhanced CT demonstrates aortic pseudoaneurysm (black arrow) with focal intimal disruption (white arrows) and periaortic edema and hemorrhage. (Courtesy of Don Yandow MD)

- o Abrupt change of aortic contour
- o Extravasation of contrast
- o Intimal flap
- o Pseudocoarctation secondary to diminished caliber descending aorta
- o May require multiplanar reformatting
  - ▪ Acquire using thin sections for CTA
  - ▪ Use rapid IV contrast bolus (2-5 cc/sec for 100-150 cc)

MR Findings
- Generally not used in acute setting
- MR angiography may be used for equivocal cases

Echocardiography Findings
- Newer techniques in transesophageal echocardiogram (TEE) are accurate
  - o Proximal ascending and descending aorta may be seen
  - o May be performed at bedside

Angiography Findings
- Classically was gold standard but recent advances in CTA have led to limited role of routine angiography
- Rupture with extravasation of contrast material
- Intimal flap (5-10%)
- Posttraumatic dissection (11%)
- Technique
  - o At least two views optimal, prefer AP, lateral, and 45° lateral anterior oblique (LAO)
  - o Rate 30 cc/sec for total volume 60 cc
  - o Consider brachial approach if possible

Imaging Recommendations
- Initial study chest x-ray then consider CECT unless urgent surgery required due to unstable clinical status

Traumatic Aortic Laceration

Differential Diagnosis
Ductus Diverticulum
- Located at aortic isthmus in 10% of normal population
- Smooth contour with obtuse margin

Penetrating Atherosclerotic Ulcer
- Location usually not at inner aspect of aortic isthmus
- Look for associated calcified atherosclerotic plaque

Pathology
General
- General path comments
  - Shear stress at points of maximal fixation of aorta
  - Laceration most often transverse
  - All layers of aortic wall involved in only 40%
- Epidemiology
  - Fall from great heights
  - Rapid deceleration

Gross Pathologic, Surgical Features
- Intimal tear with mediastinal hematoma

Clinical Issues
Presentation
- Exsanguination before reaching hospital (85% of total)
- Chest pain
- Dyspnea
- Dysphagia
- Hypertension upper extremities secondary to traumatic coarctation
- Bilateral femoral pulse deficits
- Systolic murmur in second left parasternal interface

Natural History
- 15-20% initial survival rate
- May develop chronic posttraumatic pseudoaneurysm
  - Defined as present > 3 months
  - Incidence: 2-5% patients surviving aortic transection > 24-48 hr
  - Most commonly at level of ligamentum arteriosum
- Incomplete rupture (15% of total)
  - Progression to complete rupture within 24 hours (50%)
  - False aneurysm formation (40-60%)

Treatment
- Surgical repair
  - Left thoracotomy with placement of interposition graft or primary anastomosis

Prognosis
- With surgery 60-70% survival rate
- Without intervention
  - 80% death within 1 hour
  - 85% death within 24 hours
  - 98% death within 10 weeks

Selected References
1. Dahnert WF: Radiology Review Manual 4th Ed, Lippincott Williams & Wilkins, Philadelphia, 513-4, 1999
2. Randall PA et al: Aneurysms of the Thoracic Aorta in Abrams' Angiography. 4th Ed., 477-83, 1997
3. Kadir S: Diagnostic Angiography, W. B. Saunders, Philadelphia, 149-56, 1986

Aortic Intramural Hematoma

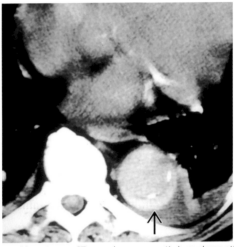

Aortic intramural hematoma. CT scan shows crescentic hyperdense attenuation in posterior aortic wall (arrow). Note displaced intimal calcifications.

Key Facts
- Synonym(s): Intramural hematoma (IMH); atypical aortic dissection
- Definition: Intramural hematoma - hemorrhage within aortic wall in absence of intimal disruption
- No intimal flap
- Descending thoracic aorta > abdominal aorta
- Hematoma formation may extend along intima
  - Results in true aortic dissection
  - True and false lumen may or may not communicate
  - Saccular aortic aneurysm may form

Imaging Findings
Classic Imaging Appearance
- Intramural hematoma: Focal aortic wall thickening without mural enhancement

Chest Radiography Finding
- Generally not seen

NECT Findings
- Acutely appears hyperdense
- Not as accurate as MRI or TEE

CECT Findings
- No enhancement within wall
- No intimal flap
- Low attenuation of aortic wall
- Suboptimal to evaluate complications
- Difficult to distinguish from
  - Dissection with thrombosed false lumen
  - Penetrating ulcer with adherent intraluminal thrombus

MR Findings
- Highly accurate
- Minimal compression of aortic lumen

Aortic Intramural Hematoma

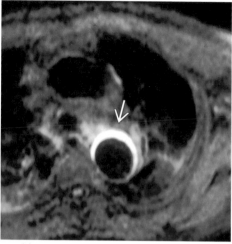

Aortic intramural hematoma. Fat-suppressed T1WI demonstrates high signal associated with subacute thrombus (arrow).

- Limited for critically ill patients
- T1WI
  - Focal thickening of aortic wall
  - No dissection flap
  - Hematoma signal changes with time
    - Isointense acutely
    - High signal subacutely
- T2WI: High signal thick wall
- Phase contrast or gadolinium may confirm lack of flow within aortic wall

Echocardiography Findings
- TEE highly accurate
- Smooth curvilinear luminal wall
- No rough irregular border (unlike penetrating ulcer)
- Homogeneous echotexture

Angiography Findings
- Intramural hematoma frequently missed
  - No intimal flap
  - No double lumen

Imaging Recommendations
- MRI or TEE best
- Multiple modalities may be required for characterization
- If MRI contraindicated or patient clinically unstable then TEE

Differential Diagnosis

Penetrating Atherosclerotic Ulcer
- Focal luminal outpouching with adjacent subintimal hematoma beneath frequently calcified and inwardly displaced intima

Saccular True Aneurysm
- Portion of aortic wall has focal bulge involving all layers
- Presence of plaque suggests penetrating atherosclerotic ulcer (PAU)

Aortic Intramural Hematoma

Mycotic Aneurysm
- Clinical symptoms help differentiate
- More inflammatory appearance
- Radiolabeled white blood cell study may differentiate

Pseudoaneurysm
- Clinical symptoms help differentiate
- More inflammatory appearance
- Adventitia of aortic wall not be well defined
- Typically located at areas of restricted aortic mobility
  - Isthmus, root, diaphragmatic hiatus

Pathology
General
- General path comments
  - 13-27% of patients clinically diagnosed with aortic dissection actually had IMH
  - IMH involves proximal aorta in approx 40%
  - IMH causes structural weakness of aortic wall
- Epidemiology
  - Common history of hypertension
  - Mean age 66 yrs; M = F
  - Lack traditional risk factors for aortic dissection

Staging Criteria
- No current formal staging criteria

Clinical Issues
Presentation
- Similar to classic aortic dissection (see Typical Aortic Dissection)

Natural History
- Intramural hematoma
  - Limited knowledge due to lack of formal evaluation
  - 33% may progress to classic dissection with intimal disruption
  - 30-40% associated with abdominal aortic aneurysm (AAA)
  - Complications
    - Occluded branch vessels: Coronary, mesenteric, renal and lower extremity arteries
    - Saccular aneurysmal enlargement of aorta
    - Aortic valve insufficiency
    - Pericardial tamponade
    - Aortic rupture

Treatment
- Lack of clinical trials to critically evaluate treatment options
- Currently empirically treated similar to typical aortic dissection

Prognosis
- Lack of clinical trials to evaluate prognosis
- Reported vascular catastrophes proximal > distal lesions

Selected References
1. Coady MA et al: Pathologic variants of thoracic aortic dissections. Penetrating atherosclerotic ulcers and intramural hematomas. Cardiol Clin 17(4):637-57, 2001
2. Sawhney NS et al: Aortic intramural hematoma: An increasingly recognized and potentially fatal entity. Chest 120(4):1340-6, 2001
3. Hayashi H et al: Penetrating atherosclerotic ulcer of the aorta: Imaging features and disease concept. Radiographics 20(4):995-1005, 2000

Penetrating Ulcer

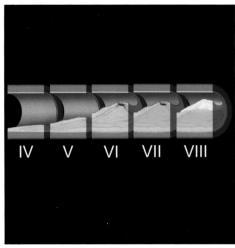

Pathologic stages of atherosclerosis. (Stages I-III not shown in figure) (I) initial atherosclerotic lesion, (II) fatty-streak, (III) preatheromic lesion, (IV) atheroma, (V) fibroatheroma, (VI) complicated lesion, (VII) calcific lesion, (VIII) fibrotic lesion.

Key Facts
- Synonym: Penetrating atherosclerotic ulcer (PAU)
- Definition: Ulcerating atherosclerotic lesion penetrates elastic lamina and forms intimal hematoma within aortic wall
- Classic imaging appearance: Focal luminal outpouching with adjacent subintimal hematoma beneath frequently calcified and inwardly displaced intima
- No intimal flap
- Descending thoracic aorta > abdominal aorta

Imaging Findings
Plain Films Findings
- Generally not seen

NECT Findings
- Requires IV contrast to visualize

CECT Findings
- Focal eccentric ulcer-like contrast collection within aortic wall
- Often associated wall thickening
- Often associated wall enhancement
- Inward displacement of frequently calcified intima
- Multiplanar reconstructions often helpful

MR Findings
- Highly accurate
- Frequently diffusely atherosclerotic aorta
- T1WI
  - Evaluation limited without gadolinium enhancement
  - Thickening of the aortic wall
- T2WI

Penetrating Ulcer

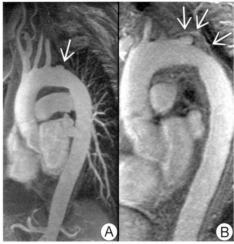

Aortic atherosclerosis with penetrating ulcer. (A) MIP image from CE-MRA shows deep ulceration at top of aortic arch (arrow). (B) Equilibrium phase sub-volume MIP demonstrates aortic atherosclerotic plaque (arrows).

- o Plaque components may be characterized on high resolution MRI, but techniques not implemented in routine clinical practice
- o T2WI show adventitia (intermediate) lipid core (dark) and cartilaginous cap (bright)
- Gd-enhanced MRA for penetrating ulcer
  - o Best with multiplanar reconstructions
  - o Eccentric ulcerlike contrast collection within aortic wall
  - o Focal associated mural enhancement

Echocardiography Findings
- Transesophageal Echocardiogram (TEE) highly accurate
- Smooth curvilinear luminal wall
- Rough irregular border
- Homogeneous echotexture

Angiography Findings
- Cross-sectional imaging required to visualize plaque
- Intra-vascular ultrasound (IVUS) may better characterize plaque

Imaging Recommendations
- No clear advantage yet described for CECT, Gd-enhanced MR, or TEE
- Evaluation without contrast is very limited

Differential Diagnosis: (PAU)

True Dissection with Thrombosed False Lumen

Intramural Hematoma

Saccular True Aneurysm
- Portion of aortic wall has focal bulge involving all layers
- Presence of plaque suggests penetrating ulcer

Mycotic Aneurysm
- Clinical symptoms help differentiate
- More inflammatory appearance
- Radiolabeled white blood cell study may differentiate

Penetrating Ulcer

Pseudoaneurysm
- Clinical symptoms help differentiate
- More inflammatory appearance
- Adventitia of aortic wall not well defined
- Typically located at areas of restricted aortic mobility
  - o Isthmus, root, diaphragmatic hiatus, graft anastomoses

Pathology
General
- Aortic atherosclerosis
  - o Classification system of Stary (see figure on previous page)
  - o Lesion types I-III mild changes that do not affect lumen
  - o Lesion types IV-VIII lesions cause arterial stenosis
- Penetrating atherosclerotic ulcer
  - o Ulcerating atherosclerotic lesion penetrates elastic lamina and forms intimal hematoma within aortic wall
    - ▪ Intracellular lipid in thickened intima
    - ▪ Extracellular lipid seen underlying intima
    - ▪ Smooth muscle proliferation
- Epidemiology
  - o Common history of hypertension
  - o PAU presents at mean age 66 yrs
  - o M = F

Clinical Issues
Presentation
- Hyperlipidemia
- Chest and back pain in setting of penetrating ulcer
Natural History
- Aortic atherosclerosis
  - o Fatty streak initially
  - o Mural thickening
  - o Some arterial remodeling early to preserve vessel lumen (Glagov Phenomenon)
  - o Late arterial stenosis and occlusion
- Penetrating atherosclerotic ulcer
  - o Limited knowledge due to lack of formal evaluation
  - o 33% may progress to classic dissection with intimal disruption
  - o 30-40% associated with abdominal aortic aneurysm (AAA)
Treatment & Prognosis (PAU)
- Atherosclerosis treated by HMG Co-A reductase inhibitors (statins)
- PAU currently empirically treated similar to typical aortic dissection
- Lack of clinical trials to evaluate prognosis
- Reported vascular catastrophes proximal > distal lesions

Selected References
1. Sawhney NS et al: Aortic intramural hematoma: An increasingly recognized and potentially fatal entity. Chest 120(4):1340-6, 2001
2. Hayashi H et al: Penetrating atherosclerotic ulcer of the aorta: Imaging features and disease concept. Radiographics 20(4):995-1005, 2000
3. Coady MA et al: Pathologic variants of thoracic aortic dissections. Penetrating atherosclerotic ulcers and intramural hematomas. Cardiol Clin 17(4):637-57, 1999

Abdominal Aortic Aneurysm

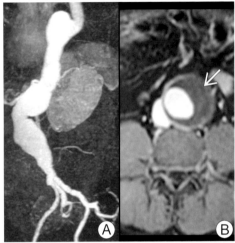

(A) CE-MRA shows abdominal aortic aneurysm (AAA). The MIP image shows branch vessel anatomy, the size of the true lumen cannot be assessed. (B) Post-contrast T1WI with fat suppression shows bright lumen of aneurysm with extensive mural thrombus (arrow). True aneurysm size is much larger than lumen diameter.

Key Facts
- Synonym(s): AAA
- Definition: Focal widening > 3cm or > 1.5x diameter of adjacent vessel
- Classic imaging appearance
  - Saccular = involvement of portion of wall
  - Fusiform = circumferential involvement
  - True aneurysm = all layers of weakened but intact walls
  - False aneurysm = focal contained perforation
- Other key facts
  - M:F = 5:1
  - Age > 60 y/o
  - Prevalence 2-3% general population
  - 91% are infrarenal
  - 66% extend into iliac arteries

Imaging Findings
CT Findings
- NECT
  - Crescent sign = peripheral high mural attenuation indicating impending rupture due to acute intramural hematoma
  - Limited to evaluate branch vessel stenosis/occlusion
  - Focal effacement of wall with retroperitoneal fluid may represent rupture
- CECT
  - Depicts luminal thrombus (80%) and branch vessel stenoses
  - Active leak depicted as extraluminal contrast
Ultrasound Findings
- 98% accurate in size measurement
- Limited evaluation of branch vessels

Abdominal Aortic Aneurysm

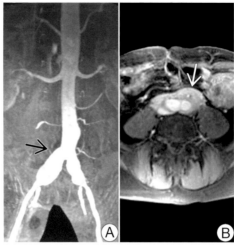

Inflammatory aneurysm with retroperitoneal fibrosis (RPF). (A) MIP image from CE-MRA shows aneurysm involving distal aorta and iliac arteries (black arrow). (B) Post-contrast fat-suppressed T1WI shows classic RPF (arrow) that characteristically spares the posterior aortic wall.

- May not visualize entire abdominal aorta in some patients

Other Modality Findings
- Plain x-ray: Mural calcification 86%
- Angio: Normal sized lumen secondary to mural thrombus in 11%
- Gd-enhanced MRA is comparable to CECT
- IMA and lumbar arteries occluded in 80%

Imaging Recommendations
- Cross-sectional imaging required to accurately depict size of aneurysm
- Must define proximal and distal extent for intervention

Differential Diagnosis

Atherosclerotic
- Etiology in approx 75%
- 29% of infrarenal aneurysms associated with thoracic aneurysm

Mycotic
- 3% of all AAAs
- Usually secondary to hematogenous spread of bacterial infection
- Saccular eccentric rapidly enlarging structure

Inflammatory
- Retroperitoneal fibrosis with smooth, enhancing rind of soft tissue around anterior and lateral aorta
- Thought to be autoimmune phenomena with transmural aortic leakage of antigen
- Idiopathic in 2/3
- Causes include NSAIDs, ergot-derivative drugs, retroperitoneal hemorrhage, desmoplastic response to tumor

Abdominal Aortic Aneurysm

Pathology

General

- General path comments
  - Increased predisposition in connective tissue and ateritis, i.e., Marfan's, Ehlers-Danlos, Takayasa's arteritis, Reiter's syndrome
- Etiology-Pathogenesis
  - Increasing lateral hydrostatic pressure as velocity of blood flow decreases leading to compromise of mural vascular nutrition
- Epidemiology
  - Elderly M > F

Gross Pathologic, Surgical Features

- True aneurysm all layers of aortic wall intact
- False (pseudo) aneurysm disruption of intima with contained rupture

Microscopic Features

- Diseased intima with secondary degeneration and fibrous replacement of media

Clinical Issues

Presentation

- Asymptomatic approx. 1/3
- Abdominal pain approx. 1/3
- Abdominal mass approx. 1/3

Natural History

- Growth rate for aneurysms 3-6 cm diameter is 0.39 cm/year
- Complications
  - Rupture (5-7 cm = 25%, 7-10 cm = 50%)
  - Spontaneous occlusion
  - Peripheral embolization
  - Infection

Treatment

- Treatment recommended for diameter > 5 cm
- Open surgical repair vs endovascular stent-graft

Prognosis

- 64-94% of ruptures die outside hospital
- Increased risk of rupture
  - Size > 6 cm
  - Growth rate > 5 mm/six months
  - Symptomatic

Selected References
1. Valji K et al: Vascular and Interventional Radiology. W.B. Saunders, Philadelphia, PA 82-91, 1999
2. Dahnert WF: Radiology Review Manual. 4th Ed., Lippincott Williams & Wilkins, Philadelphia, 506-509, 1998
3. Crawford E et al: Abdominal aortic aneurysm. N Engl J Med 321:1040-3, 1989

Infected Aortic Graft

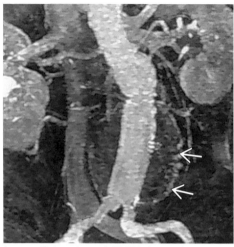

MIP image from equilibrium phase of CE-MRA shows enhancement of aortic wall (arrows). No pseudoaneurysm or graft leak is noted. (See figure on next page).

Key Facts
- Synonym(s): Postoperative graft infection or infected pseudoaneurysm
- Definition: Infection of aortic prosthetic graft
- Classic imaging appearance: Perigraft fluid, soft-tissue density, or ectopic gas beyond four weeks after surgery
- Other key facts
  - Incidence = 1-2% of all postoperative aortic graft patients
  - Graft infection is 3x more common if graft is ruptured preoperatively
  - Most common organism is staphylococcus epidermis
  - Hematoma following graft placement should resolve within 3 months of surgery

Imaging Findings
General Features
- Best imaging clue: Perigraft fluid, soft-tissue mass, or ectopic gas increasing or persisting months after graft placement
CT Findings
- NECT: Ectopic perigraft gas that is persistent or is increasing in amount over time
- CECT
  - Leakage of contrast into infectious pseudoaneurysm
  - Extensive perigraft inflammatory enhancement
MR Findings
- T1WI: Extensive perigraft soft-tissue mass, increasing over time
- T2WI: Increasing perigraft fluid collection beyond expected time of resolution (3 months)
- Contrast-enhanced MRA
  - Leakage of gadolinium contrast into infected pseudoaneurysm
  - Extensive contrast-enhancement of perigraft inflammatory mass

Infected Aortic Graft

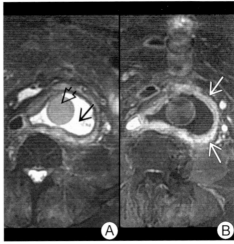

Graft infection (A) T2WI shows high-signal fluid (black arrow) around aortic graft (open arrow), a non-specific finding early after graft placement. (B) T1WI post-contrast shows marked enhancement of aortic wall due to infection (arrows).

Other Modality Findings
- Conventional x-ray angiography may be helpful for preoperative planning, although role is now smaller
- Nuclear medicine indium-111 tagged white blood cell scan may be very helpful for documenting infection

Imaging Recommendations
- Unenhanced and enhanced CT or MR
- MRA, CTA, or conventional angiography is very helpful to establish the status of vessels distal to the graft, for possible secondary repair (i.e., axillary-femoral bypass procedure)

Differential Diagnosis

Anastomotic Pseudoaneurysm
- Caused by failure of graft repair at suture line, placing excessive tension on anastomosis
- Anastomotic pseudoaneurysms may result as a secondary complication of infection of graft

Aortoenteric Fistula
- Breakdown of graft repair with erosion of aortic contents into bowel
- Duodenum is most common location of aortoenteric fistula

Normal Postoperative Resolution of Perigraft Hematoma
- Complete resolution of hematomas should occur within 3 months
- Ectopic gas should be resorbed in 3-4 weeks

Pathology

General
- Most infections are believed to be a result of contamination from the abdominal incision
- Hematogenous seeding secondary to bacteremia may be a cause of late graft infection

Infected Aortic Graft

- Etiology-Pathogenesis
  - Most common organism is staphylococcus epidermidis

Microscopic Features
- Microbiology helpful on image-guided aspiration of perigraft fluid

Clinical Issues

Presentation
- Signs and symptoms are not specific
  - Fever
  - Abdominal pain
  - Malaise
  - Palpable mass
  - Draining sinus
- Patients may present days to years following surgery

Treatment
- Antibiotic therapy
- Resection of graft with replacement

Prognosis
- High morbidity and mortality associated with operative repair of infected graft

Selected References
1. Low RN et al: Aortoenteric fistula and perigraft infection: Evaluation with CT. Radiology 175(1):157-62, 1990
2. Auffermann W et al: Incorporation vs infection of retroperitoneal aortic grafts, MR imaging features. Radiology 172(2):359-62, 1989
3. Jarrett F et al: Experience with infected aneurysms of the abdominal aorta. Arch Surg 110:1282, 1975

Endoleak Post AAA Repair

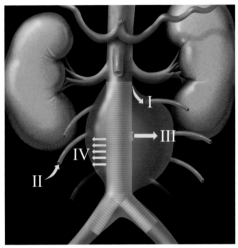

Endoleak. (I) Graft related, inadequate seal at landing zone, (II) persistent collateral flow from lumbar, inferior mesenteric branches, (III) device failure, leakage of contrast through device, fabric, at modular segments, (IV) graft porosity, now rarely seen.

Key Facts
- Definition: Persistent blood flow outside an endovascular stent graft but within an aneurysm sac
- Classic imaging appearance: Leakage of contrast material outside endograft into aneurysm sac
- Other key facts
  - Persistence of Types I and III endoleak beyond 3-6 months increases the risk of aneurysm rupture
  - Role of Type II endoleaks relative to aortic rupture is debated
  - Best surveillance method is CTA or MRA with aneurysm volume measurements

Imaging Findings
General Features
- Best imaging clue: Leakage of contrast media outside endograft into aneurysm sac
  - Broad-based leakages near prosthesis often the result of malposition of terminal end of stent graft
  - Ventral leakages without direct communication to stent graft often supplied by inferior mesenteric artery (IMA)
  - Leakages at dorsolateral aneurysm sac are often supplied by lumbar arteries
  - Large circumferential perigraft leakages indicate dislocation of stent graft or prosthesis that is too short

CT Findings
- CT is widely available, easily accessible, and well tolerated by patients
- Reproducibility of CT measures is excellent
- Delayed CT scan is important to maximize sensitivity for detecting endoleaks, but increases radiation dose

Endoleak Post AAA Repair

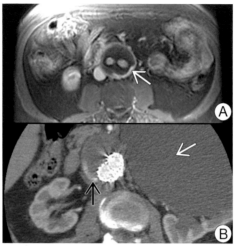

Endoleak. (A) Fat-suppressed T1WI MRI shows type II endoleak from lumbar arteries, layering along the posterior wall of aorta (arrow). (B) Axial CT from a different patient shows type III endoleak (black arrow). The endoleak developed as the cystic mass (white arrow) created discontinuity at the interface between segments.

- CT angiography is shown to be superior to intraarterial DSA for detecting endoleaks
- CT protocol
  - Pre-contrast CT as comparison for detecting small changes in contrast associated with endoleak
  - CT angiography sequence during arterial phase of contrast-enhancement
  - Delayed CT angiography sequence performed 1-2 min following contrast administration to detect late endoleak
  - CT excellent for demonstrating relationship of stent graft material to branch vessels

MR Findings
- MR protocol
  - Pre- and post-contrast fat-suppressed T1-weighted imaging for evaluation of subtle contrast enhancement
  - 3-dimensional gradient recalled echo MRA sequence before, during, 2x following injection of gadolinium contrast agent
  - Special attention is required to minimize the metal artifacts associated with the prosthesis, including short TE and large (45-90 degree) flip angle

Catheter Angiography Finding
- Role of angiography is primarily to characterize and treat endoleaks

Imaging Recommendations
- CT provides mainstay for preoperative evaluation and postoperative follow-up in aortic stent graft patients
- MRA useful in specific situations
  - Renal insufficiency
  - Allergic reactions to iodine
  - Patients with life expectancy of more than 20 years due to radiation dose associated with serial follow-up studies

- o Nitinol grafts
- o MRI not recommended in stainless steel grafts (Zenith-Cook, Endologix-Bard)

Differential Diagnosis
Type I Endoleak (Graft-Related Endoleak)
- Inadequate seal at proximal or distal landing zones of graft

Type II Endoleak (Nongraft-Related Endoleak)
- Persistent collateral blood flow into aneurysm sac flowing retrograde from
  - o Lumbar arteries, inferior mesenteric arteries, other collateral vessels

Type III Endoleak (Device Failure)
- Leakage of contrast through a defect in graft fabric
- Leakage between segments of a modular graft
- Mechanical failure of graft

Type IV Endoleak (Graft Porosity)
- Minor blush of contrast through graft material
- Seen in early phase of commercial development of stent grafts, fabric leakage is now rarely seen

Pathology
General
- General path comments
  - o Endoleak results in "endotension", persistent elevated systemic pressures in aneurysm sac
- Etiology-Pathogenesis
  - o Laplace law indicates that endotension (sac pressure) rather than flow causes expansion and rupture of aneurysm sac
- Epidemiology
  - o Eurostar registry: Endoleaks occur in 2.4-45.5% of patients following endovascular repair of thoracic and abdominal aortic aneurysms

Staging or Grading Criteria
- See Differential Diagnosis above

Clinical Issues
Presentation
- Usually asymptomatic
- Expanding aneurysm sac following endograft repair of aneurysm

Natural History
- Type I and Type III endoleaks are associated with significant risk of aneurysm rupture if left untreated
- Clinical importance of Type II endoleaks remains somewhat controversial

Treatment
- Type I and Type III endoleaks are treated with overstenting of existing graft
- Type II endoleak may be treated by embolization of lumbar or inferior mesenteric arteries, but this remains a matter of controversy

Selected References
1. Thurnher S et al: Imaging of aortic stent-grafts and endoleaks. Radiol Clin N Amer 40:799-833, 2002
2. Haulon S et al: Prospective evaluation of magnetic resonance imaging after endovascular treatment of infrarenal and aortic aneurysms. Euro J Vasc Endo Surg 22(1):62-9, 2001
3. Matsumura JS et al: Clinical consequences of periprosthetic leak after endovascular repair of abdominal aortic aneurysm. J Vasc Surg 27:606-13, 1998

Abdominal Aortic Occlusion

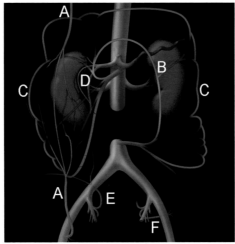

Collateral pathways in abdominal aortic occlusion: (A) Superior and inferior epigastric arteries, (B) arc of Riolan, (C) marginal artery of Drummond, (D) pancreaticoduodenal arcade, (E) iliolumbar branches, (F) superior gluteal branches.

Key Facts
- Synonym(s): Leriche syndrome
- Definition: Acute or chronic complete occlusion of the abdominal aorta
- Classic imaging appearance
  - Acute: Abrupt occlusion of abdominal aorta with filling defect
  - Chronic: Infrarenal occlusion of aorta with extensive collateral vessels
- Other key facts
  - Distal aortic occlusion propagates back toward renal arteries
  - Patient's symptoms depend on level of collateral blood flow

Imaging Findings
General Features
- Best imaging clue
  - Occlusion of infrarenal abdominal aorta +/- collateralization
MR Findings
- Contrast-enhanced MR angiography
  - Acute occlusion
    - Abrupt termination of abdominal aorta
    - Filling defect/meniscus indicating embolus
  - Chronic occlusion
    - Infrarenal occlusion of aorta with collateral filling of distal vessels
    - Reconstitutes at iliac or common femoral arteries
CT Findings
- Similar to MR angiography
- Extensive aortic calcification
Other Modality Findings
- X-ray digital subtraction angiography
  - Limited role with development of less invasive techniques (MRA, CT)
  - Vascular access difficult in absence of conduit for placement of catheter via femoral arteries

Abdominal Aortic Occlusion

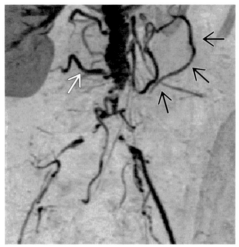

Infrarenal aortic and proximal iliac occlusion. Note the large Arc of Riolan (black arrows) and lumbar collateral artery (white arrow).

- ▪ Brachial artery approach
- ▪ Translumbar approach
- o Increased risk of complications associated with translumbar and brachial approaches

Differential Diagnosis
Chronic Aortic Occlusion Associated with Atherosclerosis
- Extensive development of collateral network
- Level of occlusion evenly distributed above and below inferior mesenteric artery
- Tendency to propagate back toward renal arteries
Aortic Embolism
- Usually large embolus from cardiac source
- Tumor embolus in setting of malignancy
Aortic Dissection
- Unusual complication of aortic dissection
- Occlusion of true lumen by enlarging false lumen
Coarctation Syndromes
- Neurofibromatosis
- William's syndrome
- Congenital rubella
- Tuberous sclerosis
- Takayasu's arteritis

Pathology
General
- General path comments
  - o Most common cause of aortic occlusion is thrombosis superimposed on severe aortic atherosclerosis

Abdominal Aortic Occlusion

- Embryology-Anatomy
  - o Development of collateral pathway is important
  - o Pancreaticoduodenal arcade (celiac to superior mesenteric artery (SMA))
  - o Arc of Riolan (SMA to inferior mesenteric artery (IMA))
  - o Marginal artery of Drummond (SMA to IMA)
  - o Iliolumbar collaterals (lumbar arteries to internal iliac branches)
  - o Superior to inferior epigastric arteries
  - o Gluteal collaterals
- Etiology-Pathogenesis
  - o See "Penetrating Ulcer"
- Epidemiology
  - o Acute abdominal aortic occlusion: Estimated 50% of cases due to embolism
  - o Chronic aortic occlusion: Elderly, history of atherosclerosis
    - ▪ Males > females
    - ▪ Smoking history

Gross Pathologic, Surgical Features
- Severe aortic atherosclerosis, calcification

Microscopic Features
- See "Penetrating Ulcer"

Clinical Issues

Presentation
- Acute occlusion
  - o Sudden onset bilateral extremity pain
  - o Absent pulses
  - o Cool skin
  - o Neurologic defects
  - o History of myocardial infarction or cardiac arrhythmia
- Chronic occlusion
  - o Leriche syndrome (described in young males in 1950)
    - ▪ Lower extremity weakness without claudication
    - ▪ Global atrophy of lower extremities with trophic changes in nails or skin
    - ▪ Delayed wound healing
    - ▪ Absence of femoral or lower extremity pulses
    - ▪ Persistent foot or leg pallor
    - ▪ Vasculogenic impotence

Treatment
- Aorto-bi-iliac graft for distal occlusion reconstituting at level of iliac arteries
- Aorto-bifemoral graft for aortic occlusion reconstituting at femoral arteries
- Axillary-femoral graft

Prognosis
- Acute aortic occlusion: > 50% mortality rate
- Chronic aortic occlusion: Significantly lower morbidity and mortality rates compared to acute aortic occlusion

Selected References
1. Ruehm SJ et al: Contrast-enhanced MR angiography in patients with aortic occlusion (Leriche syndrome). J Magn Reson Imag 11(4):401-10, 2000
2. Boender AC et al: An attempt to classify the collateral systems in total occlusions at different levels of the lumbar aorta and pelvic arteries: Causes and consequences. Radiol Clin N Amer 46:348-63, 1997

Chronic Mesenteric Ischemia

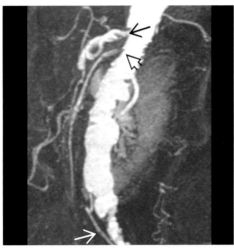

Sagittal MIP form CE-MRA exam. Celiac stenosis (black arrow) and severe superior mesenteric artery stenosis (open arrow) are demonstrated. Note severe aortic atherosclerosis and small but patent inferior mesenteric artery (white arrow).

Key Facts
- Synonym(s)
  - Abdominal angina
  - Intestinal angina
- Definition: Insufficient blood flow to the gut to satisfy needs after meals
- Classic imaging appearance: Stenosis or occlusion of at least two of the three mesenteric arteries associated with classic symptoms of abdominal pain, weight loss, and avoidance of food
- Identification of mesenteric artery occlusive disease alone does not indicate mesenteric ischemia

Imaging Findings
General Features
- Best imaging clue: Stenosis or occlusion of at least two of three mesenteric arteries
CECT Findings
- Useful for demonstrating mesenteric artery stenosis
- Role somewhat limited, patients frequently have associated renal insufficiency therefore driving diagnostic study towards MRA
MR Findings
- T1WI: Useful for excluding other causes of abdominal pain
- Contrast-enhanced MRA: Method of choice for characterizing mesenteric artery stenotic disease
  - Significant aortic atherosclerosis, especially at ostia of mesenteric arteries
  - Stenosis or occlusion of at least two of three mesenteric arteries
  - Evidence of collateral circulation
    - Pancreaticoduodenal arcade (celiac to superior mesenteric artery (SMA))
    - Arc of Riolan (SMA to inferior mesenteric artery (IMA))
    - Marginal artery of Drummond (SMA to IMA)

Chronic Mesenteric Ischemia

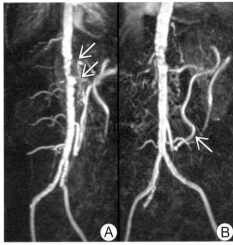

Mesenteric ischemia. (A) Note occlusion of the celiac and superior mesenteric arteries (arrows). (B) Celiac and mesenteric vessels are filled retrograde from the prominent inferior mesenteric artery through the arc of Riolan (arrow).

- Phase-contrast flow measurements: Blunted SMA flow increase 30 minutes after meal
- Mesenteric venous oxygen measurements
  - Blood oxygen level dependent imaging (use T2 measurements to infer oxygen saturation)
  - Postprandial blood oxygenation reduced in setting of chronic mesenteric ischemia

Other Modality Findings
- Conventional arteriography: Remains gold standard, however invasive, and increased risk of catheter-induced complications in these patients with extensive aortic atherosclerosis

Differential Diagnosis
Median Arcuate Ligament Syndrome
- Extrinsic compression of celiac artery by median arcuate ligament
- Controversial diagnosis as cause of abdominal pain
- Classic imaging appearance
  - Impression along superior aspect of celiac artery
  - Worse on expiration compared to inspiration
Mesenteric Thrombosis
- Chronic venous thrombosis of superior mesenteric vein may present as chronic mesenteric ischemia
- Requires use of arterial and venous phase imaging when evaluating patients with suspected mesenteric ischemia
Mesenteric Ischemia due to Other Causes
- Aortic dissection with occlusion or stenosis of mesenteric artery origins
- Vasculitis
- Vasoactive drugs causing vasoconstriction
- Fibromuscular dysplasia
- Aortic coarctation syndromes

Chronic Mesenteric Ischemia

Pathology

<u>General</u>
- General path comments
  - o Atherosclerosis of mesenteric branches is relatively frequent, but chronic mesenteric ischemia is relatively uncommon
  - o Two-thirds of patients 80 years of age and older have significant stenoses of mesenteric arteries
- Embryology-anatomy: See "Abdominal Aortic Occlusion" for description of collateral pathways
- Etiology-Pathogenesis
  - o Stenotic or occlusive disease of mesenteric arterial supply
  - o Reduced total mesenteric blood flow, incapable of keeping up with demand following meals
- Epidemiology
  - o F > M
  - o 77% of individuals older than 45 years of age have evidence of atherosclerosis

<u>Gross Pathologic, Surgical Features</u>
- Atherosclerosis involving aorta, ostia, and proximal mesenteric arteries
- Dense calcification of aortic wall

<u>Microscopic Features</u>
- Classic atherosclerotic features (see "Penetrating Ulcer")

Clinical Issues

<u>Presentation</u>
- Chronic postprandial abdominal pain
- Fear of food
- Weight loss
- Nausea
- Diarrhea
- Abdominal bruit is common but nonspecific finding in chronic mesenteric ischemia

<u>Treatment and Prognosis</u>
- Surgery is preferred and most durable form of therapy
  - o Transaortic thromboendarterectomy
  - o Aorto-mesenteric bypass
  - o Mesenteric reimplantation (distal aorta or iliac arteries)
- Percutaneous therapy
  - o Significant catheter-induced complications occur relatively frequently (up to 30%)
  - o Technical success rate is variable (30-90%)
  - o Acceptable alternative to surgery in patients at high risk for operative complications

Selected References
1. Hagspiel KD et al: MR angiography of the mesenteric vasculature. Radiol Clin N Amer 40:867-86, 2002
2. Meaney JF et al: Gadolinium-enhanced MR angiography of visceral arteries in patients with suspected chronic mesenteric ischemia. J Magn Reson Imag 7:171-6, 1997
3. Matsumoto AH et al: Percutaneous transluminal angioplasty of visceral artery stenoses: Results and long-term clinical follow-up. J Vasc Int Radiol 6:165-9, 1995

Renal Artery Stenosis

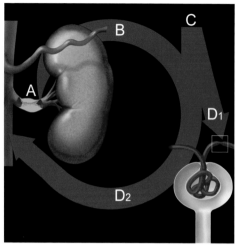

(A) Renal artery stenosis creates hypoperfusion of distal renal artery. (B) Juxtaglomerular apparatus triggers production of renin, which catalyzes. (C) Conversion of angiotensinogen to (D) angiotensin II. Angiotensin II acts as potent vasoconstrictor of efferent arteriole (D1) & causes systemic vasoconstriction (D2).

Key Facts
- Synonym(s): Renovascular hypertension; ischemic nephropathy;
- Definition: Renal artery stenosis (RAS) causing renovascular hypertension or renal insufficiency
- Classic imaging appearance
  - Single or bilateral stenosis of renal artery
  - Proximal: Atherosclerotic; distal: Fibromuscular dysplasia
- Other key facts
  - Triggers hypertension through renin-angiotensin system
  - Causes an estimated 1% of hypertension
  - Up to 15% of patients presenting for dialysis have RAS

Imaging Findings
General Features
- Focal stenosis exceeding 60% diameter
  - Ostial or proximal stenosis implies atherosclerotic RAS
  - Mid or distal stenosis implies fibromuscular dyplasia
Cross-Sectional Imaging Findings
- CECT
  - Role limited in patients with significant renal insufficiency
  - Helical CT: Sensitivity => 90%, specificity => 90%
MRA Findings
- CEMRA findings same as CT
- Sensitivity => 90%, specificity => 90%
- Phase-contrast flow measurements: Tardus-parvus flow pattern
- Signal loss on 3D phase contrast implies hemodynamically significant stenosis
Other Modality Findings
- Ultrasound

Renal Artery Stenosis

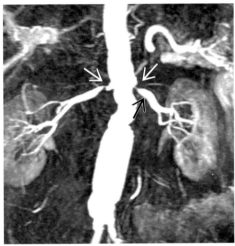

Severe bilateral renal artery stenosis (white arrows). Note post-stenotic dilatation on right (black arrow), which implies that the stenosis is hemodynamically significant. Also note infrarenal aortic aneurysm.

- o Demonstration of main renal arteries difficult
- o Doppler analysis of segmental renal flow pattern
  - ▪ Tardus-Parvus waveform associated with RAS
  - ▪ Nonspecific in patients with nephrosclerosis, high renal resistance
- Renal vein renin sampling
  - o Normal ratio of right ventricle (RV) to inferior vena cava (IVC) renin: 1.2
  - o Ratio between stenotic and normal arteries > 1.5 implies significant stenosis
- ACE inhibited renal scintigraphy
  - o Accurate in young hypertensive patient population
  - o Limited accuracy in setting of bilateral RAS or renal failure
  - o May be helpful for determining hemodynamic significance of RAS
- Digital subtraction angiography
  - o Remains gold standard for diagnosis due to high resolution
  - o Measurement of pressure gradient exceeding 15 mmHg implies hemodynamic significance of RAS

Imaging Recommendations
- Contrast-enhanced MRA for initial screening
- Confirmatory angiography and imaging for percutaneous therapy

Differential Diagnosis
Atherosclerotic RAS
- Proximal renal artery stenosis
- Ostial lesions most often atherosclerotic and may require stenting
- Diffuse renal parenchymal loss with cortical scarring
Fibromuscular Dysplasia
- Classic appearance of "string of beads": Renal stenosis with intervening aneurysm

Renal Artery Stenosis

Other Etiologies
- Vasculitis
  - o Takayasu's
  - o Polyarteritis nodosa
- Coarctation syndromes
  - o Neurofibromatosis
  - o William's syndrome
- Renal artery dissection
- Extrinsic compression: Trauma, mass

Pathology
General
- Embryology-Anatomy
  - o Prevalence of patients with accessory renal arteries is 25-35%
  - o Renal vein anomalies in 15% of patients
- Etiology-Pathogenesis (see illustration)
- Epidemiology
  - o RAS causes an estimated 1% of hypertension
  - o RAS is a significant contribution factor in an estimated 5-15% of patients presenting for dialysis

Clinical Issues
Presentation
- Renovascular hypertension should be considered in the following settings
  - o Newly onset hypertension in patients < 20 yrs or > 50 yrs
  - o Poorly controlled hypertension despite medical therapy
  - o Onset of renal insufficiency following ACE inhibition
  - o Hypertension associated with known atherosclerotic vascular disease
  - o Abdominal bruit
Treatment
- Percutaneous therapy
  - o Angioplasty for single nonostial lesions
  - o Stent placement for ostial lesions or failed angioplasty
- Surgical revascularization
  - o RAS with co-existing aortic disease requiring surgery
  - o In setting of occlusion of renal artery
Prognosis
- Renal salvage more likely successful
  - o Renal length exceeding 7 cm
  - o Renal biopsy demonstrating functional glomeruli
  - o Renal function demonstrated by nuclear scintigraphy
- Percutaneous therapy
  - o Technical success rate 80-95%
  - o Clinical improvement
    - ▪ Atherosclerosis 70%
    - ▪ Fibromuscular dysplasia (FMD) 90%
    - ▪ Renal salvage in ischemic nephropathy 50%

Selected References
1. Grist TM: Renal magnetic resonance angiography: An update. Current Opinions in Urology 8:105-9, 1998
2. Working Group on Renovascular Hypertension: Detection, evaluation, and treatment of renovascular hypertension. Arch Intern Med 147:820, 1987

Fibromuscular Dysplasia (FMD)

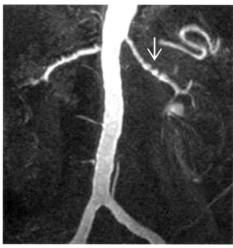

Fibromuscular dyplasia medial fibroplasia subtype. Note the "string-of-beads" appearance (arrow) due to alternating stenosis with focal aneurysms. Also note mid and distal renal artery involvement, on contrast – MRA.

Key Facts
- Pathologic condition classically resulting in areas of narrowing (stenosis) and dilatation (aneurysms) of small and medium sized arteries
- Typically involves mid and distal arteries
  - Versus atherosclerosis (typically ostial and proximal)
- Most commonly involves renal and internal carotid arteries
- Consider in all cases of hypertension under 40 years old, especially females

Imaging Findings
General Features
- Most common pathologic form demonstrates alternating areas of focal stenosis and aneurysmal dilatation of mid and distal medium and small arteries
  - "String of beads" in most common pathologic form: Medial fibroplasia
  - Most commonly affects renal or internal carotid arteries
    - Less commonly affects vertebral, subclavian, brachial, iliac, and visceral arteries
    - Coronary involvement extremely rare
CTA/MRA Findings
- Sensitivity and specificity currently unknown
- May see areas of stenosis, aneurysm, or end organ ischemic injury/ atrophy
- Normal exam does not exclude arterial dysplasia of segmental renal arteries
  - Recommend conventional arteriogram if arterial dysplasia clinically suspected
  - CTA/MRA may be used to follow for potential complications (aneurysm, dissection)

Fibromuscular Dysplasia (FMD)

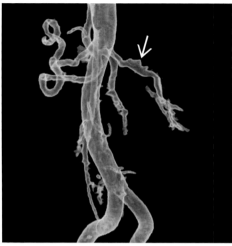

Renal aneurysm due to FMD. Note the aneurysmal enlargement of the distal left renal artery (arrow) on transparent volume-rendered CE-MRA. MRA may be used to follow renal artery aneurysm, which are at increased risk of rupture if they exceed 2 cm diameter.

Imaging Recommendations
- Conventional angiography remains the gold standard and imaging modality of choice
  - Highest resolution results in highest sensitivity and specificity
  - CTA or MRA may be used to identify disease involving larger vessels (i.e., carotid or main renal arteries)

Differential Diagnosis
Atherosclerosis
- Usually ostial or proximal main artery
Post Traumatic
- History of trauma or iatrogenic etiology
Thromboembolic and Thrombus Formation
- Usually different patient population (older or with cardiac arrhythmia)
- Focal lesion with acute onset
Vasculitis
- Clinical presentation different
  - Fever, elevated ESR, leukocytosis, additional symptoms, etc.
- Inflammatory change on biopsy
- Usually not limited to small/medium sized arteries

Pathology
General
- Non-inflammatory, non-atherosclerotic involvement of medium and small sized arteries
  - Most commonly involving renal arteries
  - Proximal one-third of the main renal artery is usually spared with involvement of middle and distal thirds
  - Bilateral renal artery involvement in 40-70%

Fibromuscular Dysplasia (FMD)

- Six pathologic types described based on which portion of arterial wall involved
  - Medial fibroplasia (60-70%)
    - Most common renal and carotid arterial dysplasia
    - Tends to occur in 25-50 year old women
    - Most commonly present with "string-of-beads" appearance
    - Aneurysms bulge beyond expected diameter of renal artery
    - Rarely progressive after age 40
  - Perimedial fibroplasia (10-15%)
    - Aneurysms do not bulge beyond diameter of renal artery
    - Narrow "string of beads"
    - Often progressive with ischemic renal atrophy
  - Medial hyperplasia (5 %)
    - Described in renal arteries, often progressive
    - Narrowing is frequently localized
  - Medial dissection (5 %)
    - Described in renal arteries, appearance of arterial dissection
    - Most frequently in younger age group
  - Intimal fibroplasia (5 %)
    - Renal arteries, but also carotid, mesenteric, and extremity arteries
    - Often progressive
  - Adventitial fibroplasia (< 1%)
    - Diffuse arterial narrowing of renal arteries
- Etiology-Pathogenesis: Idiopathic
- Epidemiology
  - F:M = 3:1
  - 30-50 yrs most common but any age can be affected
  - 20% of hypertension in children; 2-5% of hypertension in adults

Microscopic Features
- Location of fibroplasia within arterial wall determines pathologic subtype
- No sign of inflammatory vasculitis

Clinical Issues

Presentation
- Renovascular hypertension, deteriorating renal function, stroke, TIA, abdominal angina
- Classic presentation: Young female with hypertension or stroke

Natural History
- Often not detected until irreversible damage to involved organ

Treatment
- Medical therapy: Hypertension should be medically managed
- Data supports conventional angioplasty in renal and carotid disease
  - Up to 90% long term success rates with balloon angioplasty
  - Stents are avoided to prevent interference with possible surgery
- Surgical treatment reserved for failed percutaneous treatment

Selected References
1. Brant EW et al: Fundamentals of Diagnostic Radiology. 2nd Edition. 593-603, 1999
2. Fauci SA et al: Harrison's Principles of Internal Medicine. 14th Edition. 1400, 2341, 1998
3. Baum S: Abrams' Angiography. 4th Edition. 307-11, 1250-7, 1997

Polyarteritis Nodosa (PAN)

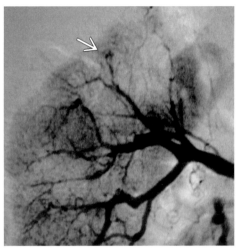

Polyarteritis nodosa. Digital subtraction angiogram demonstrates microaneurysms (arrow) as well as multiple occlusions of segmental and subsegmental renal arteries, classic findings in PAN.

Key Facts
- Noninfectious necrotizing vasculitis
  - Involvement restricted to small or medium muscular arteries
- Renal and visceral vessels most commonly involved pulmonary circulation usually spared
  - Impaired perfusion causes ulceration, ischemia, infarction, or hemorrhage
  - Without treatment fatal in most cases

Imaging Findings
General Features
- Aneurysms or occlusions of small and medium sized arteries
  - Most commonly affects kidneys, visceral organs, skin, coronaries, and peripheral nerves

Conventional Angiography Findings
- Imaging modality of choice: Highest sensitivity
- Characteristic findings in 60%
  - Smooth arterial stenosis with fusiform or saccular aneurysms
  - Multiple micro-aneurysms considered pathognomonic in patients with clinical picture of PAN

MRI/CTA Findings
- Poor sensitivity secondary to less resolution make MRI and CTA poor imaging choices for identifying arterial pathology
- May see end organ damage including infarction, intraparenchymal hemorrhage

Imaging Recommendations
- Conventional angiography remains imaging modality of choice

Polyarteritis Nodosa (PAN)

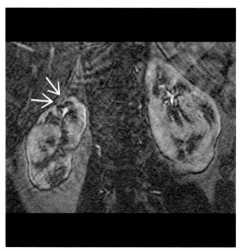

MRI image of kidneys demonstrate cortical thinning associated with segmental occlusion and parenchymal infarction (arrows).

Differential Diagnosis

Allergic Angiitis and Granulomatosis (Churg-Strauss disease or Microscopic polyangiitis)
- Histologically similar to PAN except
  - Has a high frequency of lung involvement
    - Strong association with severe asthma
  - Involves vessels of various types and sizes peripheral eosinophilia common

Pathology

General
- Definitive diagnosis by biopsy of involved organ
  - Biopsy of symptomatic organ up to 70% sensitive
  - Biopsy of asymptotic organ approximately 30% sensitive
- Spares pulmonary circulation
- Neither glomerulonephritis nor vasculitis of arterioles, capillaries, or venules is present
- Etiology-Pathogenesis
  - Immunologic mechanism
    - Noninfectious
    - Some cases thought to be complication of hepatitis B or C infection
    - Other rare associations with HIV, CMV, Parvo B19, streptococcus infection
- Epidemiology
  - Classically young and middle aged adults, although can affect children and older adults; male to female (1.6:1.0)
  - Rare with prevalence of 6.3 per 100,000 in U.S.A.

Gross Pathologic, Surgical Features
- Individual lesions involve sharply localized segments of a vessel with a predilection for branching points and bifurcations

Polyarteritis Nodosa (PAN)

- Intravascular thrombosis is a frequent sequela to acute vasculitis
- Impaired perfusion causes ulceration, ischemic atrophy, infarcts, or localized hemorrhage

Microscopic Features
- Three microscopic stages
  - Acute: Fibrinoid necrosis of the arterial wall
  - Healing: Transmural scarring with necrosis
  - Healed: Replacement with fibrous tissue

Clinical Issues

Presentation
- Clinical presentation can be puzzling with multiple different organ systems involved
- Most common signs and symptoms
  - Fever of unknown origin
  - Weight loss
  - Hypertension (rapid onset common)
  - Vasculitic skin lesions (palpable purpura, livedo reticularis, digital gangrene, or tender nodules)
  - Abdominal pain, melena
- May be acute, subacute, or chronic
  - Onset frequently gradual in onset over weeks to months
  - Frequently remittent, with long symptom free intervals
- Presents at any age although classically young and middle aged adults
  - Rare in the very young
- ESR (usually > 60 mm/hour) almost always elevated

Diagnosis
- Single biopsy followed by angiography reported sensitivity of 85% and 96% specificity

Natural History
- Usually fatal without treatment within 2 to 5 years
  - Either with an acute fulminant attack or following a protracted course

Treatment & Prognosis
- Corticosteroids and Cyclophosphamide traditional therapy
- With proper treatment remission or cure in up to 90% with classic PAN
  - 10-year survival of 70%
  - Most common causes of death include GI hemorrhage, chronic heart failure, and infection

Selected References
1. Schoen FJ et al: Blood Vessels in Robbins Pathologic Basis of Disease. 6th ed. W.B. Saunders Co., Philadelphia. 520-1, 1999
2. Fauci S et al: Harrison's Principles of Internal Medicine. 14th Ed., McGraw-Hill, New York, 1910-4, 1998
3. Cross III DT et al: Abnormalities of Cerebral Vessels in Abrams' Angiography 4th Ed. Baum S., Editor. Little, Brown and Company, Boston. 305-7, 1997

Iliac Stenosis and Occlusion

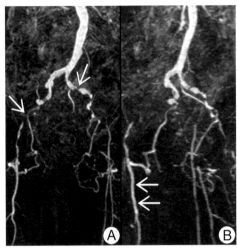

Bilateral severe iliac stenosis and occlusion. (A) A-P projection from CE-MRA shows severe iliac stenosis and occlusions (arrows). (B) Oblique MIP demonstrates reconstitution of common femoral circulation (arrows) through multiple collaterals.

Key Facts
- Definition: Inflow vessel stenosis or occlusion
- Classic imaging appearance
  - Arterial stenoses usually at bifurcations
  - Presence of collateral flow implies chronicity
  - Irregular narrowing suggests atherosclerosis
  - Smooth, abrupt bifurcation occlusions suggest embolism
  - Post-stenotic dilatation distal to severe chronic stenoses
  - Severe stenosis may progress to complete occlusion
    - Thrombus forms above lesion
    - May propagate into proximal patent branch vessel

Imaging Findings
Duplex Ultrasound Findings
- Useful for postoperative evaluation of femoral crossover
- Limited applicability in common iliac arteries
CTA Findings
- Peripheral CTA provides high resolution images of aortoiliac circulation
- Studies showing diagnostic accuracy only recently available
- Heavily calcified lesions may limit usefulness of rendered images, need to perform interpretation including source images
- Requires multidetector CT with high contrast dose at rapid bolus, sophisticated post-processing
MRA Findings
- Time of flight technique inaccurate due to flow-related artifacts (in-plane flow saturation, retrograde flow, tortuous vessels)
- Gadolinium-enhanced MRA nearly equivalent to conventional angiogram for aortoiliac disease when performed optimally (sensitivity, specificity > 90%)

Iliac Stenosis and Occlusion

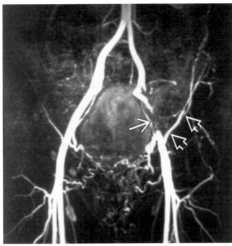

Posttraumatic left external iliac occlusion. CE-MRA shows complete occlusion of the left external iliac artery (arrow) with reconstitution of the left common femoral artery from prominent epigastric collaterals (open arrows). Patient had history of acetabular fracture with pelvic hematoma.

Angiography Findings
- Current gold standard for vessel characterization
- Minimally invasive
- Risks
  - Contrast reaction: Allergic, nephrotoxicity especially if diabetic
  - Arterial dissection
  - Pseudoaneurysm at arterial entry site

Imaging Recommendations
- Initial claudication evaluation
  - Segmental pressures or duplex ultrasound at rest
  - Consider exercise testing if normal rest exam
- If further imaging is required
  - MRA runoff if no contraindications
  - Consider CTA in patient with normal renal function
  - Conventional angiography for selected patients
    - Suboptimal MRA
    - Severely claustrophobic
    - Lesion amenable to percutaneous intervention

Differential Diagnosis

Atherosclerosis
- Irregular or eccentric narrowing, especially at posterior aspect aortic bifurcation, common iliac arteries
- Internal iliac stenosis common

Embolic Disease
- Acute or subacute symptoms
- Located at vessel bifurcations
- Lack of collateral vessels
- Search for etiology: Proximal aneurysm, cardiac vegetations

Iliac Stenosis and Occlusion

Traumatic Occlusion
- Most common cause of iliac occlusion in young, pelvic trauma, catheterization-related injury (dissection, hematoma)

Radiation Vasculitis
- Patient with history of pelvic irradiation

Neurogenic Claudication
- Neuropathy associated with severe spinal stenosis

Pathology
General
- General path comments
  - Younger patients more likely to have vasculitis, tumor encasement, or dissection
  - Older patients more likely to have atherosclerosis
- Etiology-Pathogenesis
  - Atherosclerotic intimal plaques result from smooth muscle proliferation and extracellular lipid/collagen deposition which project into the vessel lumen
- Epidemiology
  - M >> F
  - Incidence increases with age
    - 3% incidence age 45-54 yrs, 6% incidence age 55-64 yrs

Clinical Issues
Presentation
- Intermittent claudication
  - Symptoms progressively more severe with activity
  - Symptoms subside after several minutes rest
  - Graded by distance patient is able to walk
  - Location of pain may indicate level of obstruction
    - Buttock: Aorta, common iliac artery
    - Thigh: External iliac, common femoral artery
  - Impotence
    - Internal iliac artery, pudendal and obturator steal, Leriche syndrome, bilateral claudication, muscle atrophy, including thigh vasogenic impotence

Treatment
- Acute occlusive thrombus
  - Thrombolysis trial, angioplasty occasionally successful, surgical thrombectomy
- Stenosis
  - Focal (< 5 cm length)
    - Angioplasty: 92% primary patency, 69% patency at 3 yrs
    - Stents increasingly used: 97% primary patency, 80-90% patency at 5 yrs
    - Surgical revascularization (>5 cm lesion): Gold standard for long-term patency; bypass or endarterectomy; axillary/aorto/femoral

Selected References
1. Grist TM: MRA of the abdominal aorta and lower extremities. J Magn Reson Imag 11:32-43, 2000
2. Williams JE et al: Vascular Radiology in Fundamentals of Diagnostic Radiology 2nd Ed, Brant, W.E. and Helms C.A., Editors. Williams and Wilkins, Baltimore. 588-96, 1999
3. Valji K: Pelvic and lower extremity arteries. In Vascular and Interventional Radiology. W.B. Saunders, Philadelphia. 109-117, 1999

Superficial Femoral Occlusion

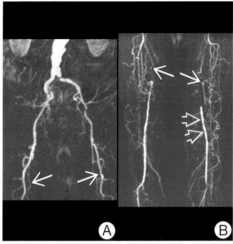

Superficial femoral artery (SFA) occlusion. CE-MRA at (A) aorto-iliac station & (B) femoral-popliteal station. (A) The images show complete occlusion of the proximal superficial femoral arteries bilaterally (arrows). (B) Note extensive profunda collaterals (arrows) and multiple stenoses in distal left SFA (open arrows).

Key Facts
- Synonym(s): SFA disease (See also discussion of Iliac Disease)
- Definition: Extremity ischemia secondary to acute or chronic arterial stenosis
- Arterial stenoses usually at bifurcations
- Presence of collateral flow implies chronicity
- Irregular narrowing suggests atherosclerosis
- Smooth abrupt bifurcation occlusions suggest embolism
- SFA disease tends to be most severe in proximal 1/3 or at adductor canal

Imaging Findings
Segmental Limb Blood Pressures
- Segmental lower extremity pressures help localize disease
  - \> 30 mmHg difference between segments is significant
- Ankle-Brachial Index (ABI)
  - Ratio of systolic ankle pressure to higher of two systolic brachial pressures
  - May be falsely elevated in diabetics with heavy calcifications
  - ABI usually correlates well with vascular insufficiency
    - ABI 0.9-1.0: Normal or minimal disease
    - ABI 0.7-0.89: Mild disease
    - ABI 0.35-0.69: Moderate disease, claudication
    - ABI < 0.3: Severe disease, limb salvage
Duplex Ultrasound Findings
- Most often used for bypass graft surveillance
  - Systolic velocity ratio > 2 at suspected stenosis
  - Peak systolic velocity < 45 cm/sec
CTA Findings
- Provides high resolution images of lower extremity circulation

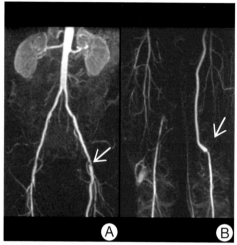

Left femoral-popliteal bypass graft stenosis. CE-MRA at (A) aortoiliac station & (B) femoral-popliteal station. (A) Stenosis at proximal anastomosis (arrow). (B) Distal anastomosis (arrow) is confirmed on MRA following Doppler ultrasound that demonstrated elevated peak systolic velocities. Note right SFA occlusion.

- Studies showing diagnostic accuracy only recently available
- Heavily calcified lesions may limit usefulness of rendered images, need to perform interpretation including source images
- Requires multi-detector CT with high contrast dose at rapid bolus

MRI/MRA Findings
- Time-of-flight technique accurate in SFA distribution, but lengthy
- Gadolinium enhanced MRA nearly equivalent to conventional angiogram for SFA disease when performed optimally (sensitivity, specificity > 90%)

Angiography Findings
- Current gold standard for vessel characterization
- Risks of contrast reaction, renal insufficiency, arterial dissection

Imaging Recommendations
- Initial claudication evaluation
  - Segmental pressures or duplex ultrasound at rest
  - Consider exercise testing if normal rest exam
- If further imaging is required
  - MRA runoff if no contraindications
  - Conventional angiography for selected patients
    - Suboptimal MRA
    - Severely claustrophobic
    - Lesion amenable to percutaneous intervention

Differential Diagnosis
Atherosclerosis
- Commonly associated with diabetes mellitus
- Increases with age
- Stenoses at bifurcations or extrinsic vascular compressions

Embolic Disease
- Acute or subacute symptoms

Superficial Femoral Occlusion

- Located at vessel bifurcations
- Lack of collateral vessels

Pathology
<u>General</u>
- General path comments
  - o Younger patients more likely to have vasculitis or entrapment
  - o Older patients more likely to have atherosclerosis
- Etiology-Pathogenesis
  - o Atherosclerotic intimal plaques result from smooth muscle proliferation and extracellular lipid/collagen deposition which project into the vessel lumen
- Epidemiology
  - o M > F
  - o Incidence increases with age
    - ▪ 3% incidence age 45-54 yrs
    - ▪ 6% incidence age 55-64 yrs

Clinical Issues
<u>Presentation</u>
- Symptoms usually reflect severity
  - o Intermittent claudication
  - o Rest pain
  - o Ulceration and gangrene
<u>Natural History</u>
- 10 yrs post initial presentation only 10% require amputation
- Eventually 25% require some type of revascularization
- 30-50% of claudicators die from coronary artery disease (CAD) or cardiovascular accident (CVA)
<u>Treatment</u>
- Surgical revascularization
  - o Gold standard for long-term patency
  - o Femoral-popliteal or distal bypass
    - ▪ Synthetic graft (Gore-Tex, Dacron)
    - ▪ Venous graft
    - ▪ Reversed saphenous
    - ▪ In situ vein graft
- Percutaneous angioplasty +/- stent
  - o Lesions < 5 cm in length
  - o Primary patency 85%
  - o Three-year patency 50%
<u>Prognosis</u>
- Four times higher rate of amputation and gangrene in diabetics

Selected References
1. Grist TM: MRA of the abdominal aorta and lower extremities. J Magn Reson Imag 11:32-43, 2000
2. Valji K: Pelvic and lower extremity arteries. In: Vascular and Interventional Radiology. W.B.Saunders, Philadelphia, 117-9, 1999

Popliteal Entrapment

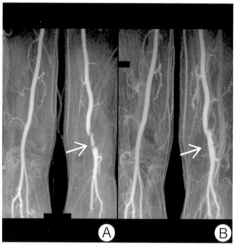

Popliteal entrapment. (A) MRA obtained during active plantar flexion demonstrates focal stenosis (arrow) of popliteal artery due to fibrous band found at surgery. (B) MRA obtained during dorsiflexion shows ectasia of popliteal artery (arrow).

Key Facts
- Synonym(s): Popliteal entrapment syndrome
- Definition: Intermittent claudication induced by compression of popliteal artery between musculoskeletal structures
- Classic imaging appearance
  - Medial deviation of the popliteal artery in the popliteal region
  - Stenosis/compression of the mid popliteal artery during prolonged plantar flexion
- Most commonly caused by compression from the medial head of the gastrocnemius muscle (74%)
- Usually presents in healthy, athletic males complaining of claudication syndrome in the absence of atherosclerosis
- Combined functional and anatomic imaging required
  - MRA or angiography in neutral position, dorsiflexion, and plantar flexion
  - MRI for anatomic definition of gastrocnemius, soleus, and popliteus muscles

Imaging Findings
General Features
- Best imaging clue: Medial deviation of popliteal artery during prolonged planter flexion with associated stenosis
CT Findings
- NECT: Limited role due to difficulty in identifying popliteal artery
- CECT
  - CTA useful for delineating the popliteal artery
  - Soft tissue contrast less well suited for demonstrating muscular anatomy than MRI
MR Findings
- T1WI: T1-weighted MRI is particularly well suited for demonstrating the anatomic variants of the gastrocnemius muscle and popliteal muscle

Popliteal Entrapment

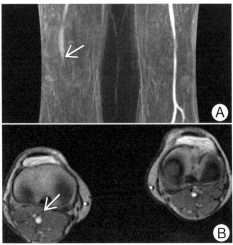

CE-MRA shows complete occlusion of right popliteal artery during plantar flexion (arrow). (B) Gradient echo image demonstrates fibrous/muscular band anterior to the right popliteal artery (arrow). Image from left leg shows normal relationship of popliteal artery and vein to gastrocnemius muscle.

- Findings include
  - Popliteal artery deviates medially around the medial head of the gastrocnemius muscle
  - Medial head of gastrocnemius muscle arises laterally from the femoral condyle
  - Popliteal artery may be trapped by a lateral slip of the medial head of the gastrocnemius muscle
  - The popliteal muscle or a deep fibrous band compresses popliteal artery
- T2WI: T2WI may be helpful for identifying and characterizing other masses that may occur in the popliteal fossa
- Contrast-enhanced MRA
  - MR angiogram in neutral position demonstrates normal artery or narrowing and medial deviation of midportion of popliteal artery
  - MRA may demonstrate post-stenotic dilatation involving popliteal artery
  - During prolonged plantar flexion, popliteal stenosis is detected

Conventional Angiography Findings
- Similar findings described above for MRA

Duplex Ultrasound Findings
- Similar findings to cross-sectional imaging; requires skilled sonographer

Imaging Recommendations
- MRI followed by contrast-enhanced MR angiography in neutral, plantar flexion, and dorsal flexion positions

Differential Diagnosis
Cystic Adventitial Disease (CAD)
- Rare condition, mucin collects in the adventitial layer of popliteal artery
- Middle-aged men with sudden onset calf pain and claudication
- MRA/angiographic appearance is of smooth, eccentric, extrinsic "hour-glass" narrowing of the popliteal artery in neutral position

Popliteal Entrapment

Popliteal Artery Aneurysm
- Patients with history of atherosclerotic and/or aneurysmal disease
- MRA/CTA/angiography demonstrates ectasia of popliteal artery

Popliteal Artery Embolism
- Abrupt onset of claudication
- Patient with history of embolic source
- Angiographic findings (MRA/CTA/angiography) demonstrate abrupt "cutoff" of popliteal artery with meniscus associated with embolus, and few collaterals

Pathology
General
- Generally regarded as congenital condition
- Etiology-Pathogenesis (see classification criteria below for mechanism)
- Epidemiology
  - Male >> female, 15:1
  - Age 12-65 years, most less than 30 years
  - Incidence unknown, estimated at 0.165% of 20,000 Greek army patients
  - Bilateral in 22-67%

Gross Pathologic, Surgical Features
- See classification criteria below

Microscopic Features
- Exam of the arterial segment demonstrates abundant longitudinal muscle fibers in the tunica media
- Internal elastic lamina is disrupted with fibrous thickening of intima

Staging or Grading Criteria
- Type I anomaly: Popliteal artery (PA) deviates medially around the medial head of the gastrocnemius muscle that arises close to its normal location
- Type II: Medial head of gastrocnemius muscle arises more laterally on femoral condyle
- Type III: PA is trapped by lateral slip of the medial gastrocnemius muscle
- Type IV: Popliteus muscle or deep fibrous band compresses PA

Clinical Issues
Presentation
- Athletic male complaining of claudication symptoms in absence of atherosclerosis
- Not unusual for onset of symptoms to be sudden
- May complain of nocturnal cramps, numbness, paresthesias
- Acute thrombosis and/or distal embolization may occur if popliteal artery shows extensive post-stenotic dilatation and aneurysm formation

Treatment
- Transection of muscle or fibrous band with mobilization of popliteal artery
- Condition of popliteal artery dictates need for vascular intervention

Prognosis
- Excellent

Selected References
1. Forester BB et al: Comparison of two-dimensional time-of-flight dynamic magnetic resonance angiography with digital subtraction angiography in popliteal artery entrapment syndrome. Can Assoc Radiol J 48:11, 1997
2. Hoelting T et al: Entrapment of the popliteal artery and its surgical management in a 20-year period. Br J Surg 84:338, 1997
3. Collins PS et al: Popliteal artery entrapment: An evolving syndrome. J Vasc Surg 10:484 1989

Acute Lower Extremity Ischemia

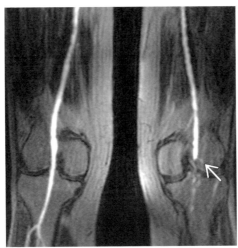

Acute popliteal occlusion. Note the abrupt termination of the left popliteal artery, with absence of collaterals (arrow). An embolus was discovered at the time of surgery.

Key Facts
- Usually caused by acute embolic or thrombotic arterial occlusion
- Most common source of emboli is cardiac
- Extent of collateral circulation determines degree of limb ischemia

Imaging Findings
<u>General Features</u>
- Best imaging clue: Abrupt termination of distal femoral or popliteal artery
<u>CT Findings</u>
- NECT: Extensive calcification in lower extremity arterial walls
- CTA: Abrupt occlusion +/- filling defect, similar findings as on MRA
<u>MR Findings</u>
- T1WI: Lack of flow void, although this sign is unreliable in lower extremity due to reversal of diastolic flow that is normal
- T2WI: May see increased soft tissue signal intensity when edema is present
- MRA
  - Embolism
    - Macroemboli usually lodged in distal femoral or popliteal artery
    - Total occlusion is seen, with presence of "meniscus" indicating embolus
    - Absence of collaterals
    - In microembolization syndromes, shaggy, ulcerated atherosclerotic disease is found in proximal vessels
  - Thrombotic occlusion
    - Presence of significant atherosclerotic disease elsewhere
    - Abrupt termination of vessel with or without collateral formation
    - Presence of popliteal aneurysm with associated thrombosis
<u>Other Modality Findings</u>
- DSA (same diagnostic findings as above)

Acute Lower Extremity Ischemia

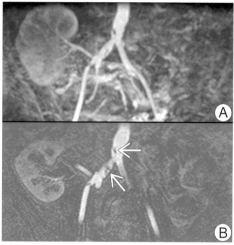

(A) MIP and (B) source images from same patient as prior image demonstrated source of embolus. Note the atherosclerotic plaque projecting into the lumen of distal aorta and common iliac artery (arrows). Note renal transplant.

- DSA (same diagnostic findings as above)
  - Remains gold standard for diagnosing and treating acute occlusion

Differential Diagnosis
Embolization
- Macroembolization
  - Cardiac source (left atrium or left ventricular thrombus)
  - Proximal atherosclerotic plaque
  - Abdominal or thoracic aortic aneurysm
- Microembolization
  - Cholesterol embolization from prior catheterization
  - Blue toe syndrome: Subacute or chronic microembolization

Acute Thrombosis
- Thrombosis due to preexisting arterial stenosis or obstruction
- Arterial bypass graft thrombosis
- Thrombosis at site of aneurysm
- Hypercoagulable state

Trauma
- Commonly associated with dislocation of the knee
- Pelvic trauma may create external iliac occlusion
- Iatrogenic (arterial catheterization)

Pathology
General
- General path comments
  - Consequences of acute arterial occlusion hinge on multiple factors
    - Degree of collateral circulation
    - Duration of occlusion and presence of oxygen-free radicals
    - Reperfusion injury
    - Tibial compartment pressure

- ▪ Cellular edema causing microvascular obstruction with "no-reflow" phenomenon
- Etiology-pathogenesis
  - o Embolic source in a majority of cases
  - o Thrombosis superimposed on chronic atherosclerotic disease

Gross Pathologic, Surgical Features

- Macroembolization: Large embolus, usually lodges at distal femoral or popliteal artery

Microscopic Features

- Microscopic embolization
  - o Atheromatous material from ulcerated plaques or aneurysms
  - o Cholesterol crystals
  - o Fibrin-platelet deposits
  - o Cellular thrombi

Staging or Grading Criteria

- Society of Vascular Surgery reporting standards for limb viability
  - o Viable: Extremity not immediately threatened
    - ▪ No rest pain or neurologic deficit
    - ▪ Skin circulation appears adequate
    - ▪ Audible Doppler flow signals
    - ▪ Ankle pressures above 30 mmHg
  - o Threatened viability: Implies reversible ischemia and a foot that is salvageable with major amputation if arterial obstruction is promptly relieved
    - ▪ Patients complain of ischemic rest pain and mild neurologic deficits
    - ▪ Audible arterial signals are not present in pedal arteries
    - ▪ Doppler venous signals are present with augmentation maneuvers
  - o Major, irreversible ischemic change: Frequently requires major amputation of limb
    - ▪ Absent capillary or skin flow
    - ▪ Profound sensory loss or muscle paralysis
    - ▪ Muscle rigor
    - ▪ Absent Doppler pulses in arterial or venous system

Clinical Issues

Presentation

- Classic presentation of "6 P's"
  - o Pain, pallor, paresthesias, pulselessness, paralysis, polar (cold) sensation

Treatment

- Percutaneous therapy enzymatic thrombolysis
- Mechanical thrombectomy
- Thromboaspiration
- Surgical therapy
  - o Fogarty balloon thromboembolectomy
  - o Bypass grafting

Selected References
1. Valji K: Acute lower extremity ischemia. In: Vascular and Interventional Radiology. W.B. Saunders, Philadelphia. 117-119, 1999
2. Comerota AJ et al: Acute arterial occlusion. In: Peripheral Vascular Diseases, 2nd edition by Young JR et al. Mosby Publishing, St. Louis. 273-87, 1996
3. Wagner HJ et al: Acute embolic occlusions of infrainguinal arteries: Percutaneous aspiration embolectomy in 102 patients. Radiology 182:403, 1992

Arterial Venous Malformation

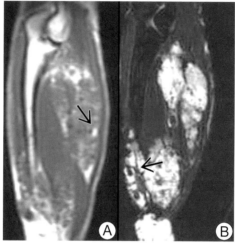

Slow flow arterial venous malformation (AVM) of the forearm. (A) T1WI shows heterogenous signal intensity due to fat within AVM (arrow). (B) T2WI shows high signal from slow flow, as well as multiple low-signal lesions from thrombus (arrow).

Key Facts
- Synonym(s): AVM
- Definition: Congenital abnormal development of network between capillaries and veins, AVMs have dysregulated angiogenesis, undergo continued vascular remodeling

Imaging Findings
General Features
- Best imaging clue: Tightly packed mass of enlarged vascular channels; best diagnostic sign = "bag of black worms" (flow voids) on spin-echo MRI
CT Findings
- NECT: Ca++ in approximately 30%
- CECT: Strong enhancement
MR Findings
- Varies with flow rate, direction, presence/age of hemorrhage
- T1WI
  - "Honeycomb" of "flow voids" in fast flow AVM
  - Foci of high signal intensity associated with fat
- T2WI
  - Very high signal intensity on fat-suppressed T2-weighted imaging if flow is slow
  - Bright "bag of worms"
- MRA
  - 3D time-resolved contrast-enhanced studies important for delineation of arterial feeders and draining veins
    - Early venous filling
    - Rapid venous washout
  - High-resolution 3D MRA useful for delineating internal architecture
Other Modality Findings
- DSA

Arterial Venous Malformation

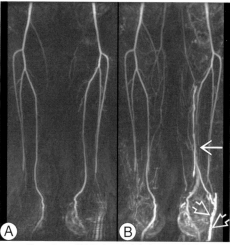

Arterial venous malformation. (A) Early arterial phase and (B) venous phase from time-resolved 3D contrast MRA shows early venous filling (arrow) from rapid flow AVM in the left foot (open arrows).

- ○ Delineates internal angio architecture (superselective best)
- ○ Numerous arterial venous connections around nidus of malformation
- ○ Early venous filling
- ○ Rapid venous washout

Differential Diagnosis
Hemangiomas
- Vascular malformation that occurs in capillary stage of development
- Benign vascular tumors, present in infancy, proliferate over time, usually involute during adulthood
- Usually cutaneous or mucosal lesion
- Also found in brain, liver, spleen, pancreas, kidneys
- Normal-caliber feeding vessels
- Early filling of vascular spaces that persist through venous phase

Arterial Venous Fistula
- Almost always acquired abnormalities
- Direct connection between artery and neighboring vein
- Usually manifestation of trauma

Pathology
General
- General path comments
  - ○ Usually associated with other syndrome
- Etiology-Pathogenesis
  - ○ Dysregulated angiogenesis
  - ○ Vascular endothelial growth factor (VEGF) receptors mediate endothelial proliferation, migration
  - ○ Cytokine receptors mediate vascular maturation, remodeling
- Epidemiology
  - ○ Prevalence of sporadic AVMs = 0.04-0.52%

Arterial Venous Malformation

Gross Pathologic, Surgical Features
- Central nidus plus arterial feeders, venous outflow

Microscopic Features
- Feeding arteries, draining veins are mature vessels
- Nidus
  - Thin-walled dysplastic vessels (no capillary bed)
  - Conglomeration of numerous AV shunts

Clinical Issues

Presentation
- Most frequently located in extremities, head, neck, and pelvis
- Painful mass
- May present with ulceration or bleeding
- In extremities, unusual to have significant shunting

Natural History
- Spontaneous obliteration is rare

Treatment
- Embolization, radiotherapy, surgery

Selected References
1. Mulliken JB et al: Vascular anomalies. Curr Prob Surg 37(8):521, 2000
2. Fellows KE: What is an arterial venous malformation? Cardvasc Intervent Radiol 10:53, 1987
3. Szilagyi DE et al: Congenital arterial venous anomalies of the limbs. Arch Surg 111:423, 1976

Arterial Venous Fistula

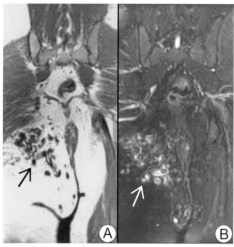

Arterial venous fistula (AVF). Spin echo images. (A) T1WI demonstrates multiple flow voids and "tangle of worms" configuration (arrow). (B) T2WI shows mostly flow void, with scattered areas of higher signal intensity, indicating that the lesion is a high flow lesion (arrow). (See next figure for MRA).

Key Facts
- Synonym(s): AVF
- Definition: Abnormal communication between an adjacent artery and vein
- Other key facts
  - Almost always acquired posttraumatic abnormalities
  - Most often occurs in extremities, where arteries and veins are adjacent to each other and near the surface
  - Marked increase in venous return to heart with associated high cardiac output and rapid heart rate, "high output failure"

Imaging Findings
General Features
- Best imaging clue: Large arterial to venous shunt with rapid transit time
CT Findings
- NECT: May see sequelae of prior trauma (foreign bodies, shrapnel)
- CECT: Strong enhancement
MR Findings
- T1WI
  - Large vessels "flow void"
  - Evidence of prior trauma
- MRA
  - Large feeder vessel
  - Enlarged, aneurysmal venous outflow
  - Rapid arterial to venous transit time
Other Modality Findings
- DSA may be used to evaluate more complex cases, including the depiction of
  - Size and number of feeder arteries
  - Collateral circulation
  - Venous circulation distal to the fistula

Arterial Venous Fistula

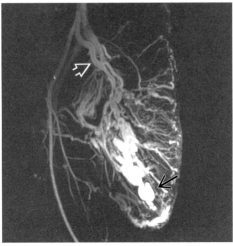

Arterial venous fistula. Contrast MRA performed with 3D time-resolved acquisitions demonstrates large AVF with arterial supply from enlarged right internal iliac artery (open arrow). Note venous aneurysms and extensive superficial and deep vein collaterals (arrow). Patient has history of penetrating right buttock trauma.

- o Possible aneurysm formation

Differential Diagnosis

Hemangiomas
- Vascular malformation that occurs in capillary stage of development
- Benign vascular tumors, present in infancy, proliferate over time, usually involute during adulthood
- Usually cutaneous or mucosal lesion
- Also found in brain, liver, spleen, pancreas and kidneys
- Normal-caliber feeding vessels
- Early filling of vascular spaces that persists through venous phase

Arterial Venous Malformation
- Congenital abnormal development of network between capillaries and veins
- Often have slower flow, therefore bright signal intensity on T2-weighted imaging, and incomplete flow void on T1-weighted imaging
- No history of trauma

Pathology

General
- General path comments
  - o Lower extremities are more frequently involved due to proximity of arteries and veins and increased likelihood for trauma
- Etiology-Pathogenesis
  - o Gunshot wound in 50% of cases
  - o Less commonly iatrogenic (disk surgery, balloon thrombectomy, percutaneous catheterization)
  - o Dialysis fistulas special case

Arterial Venous Fistula

<u>Gross Pathologic, Surgical Features</u>
- Direct communication between artery and vein
- Often have multiple arterial-venous communications
- Venous channels distal to fistula become dilated because of increased flow and direct exposure to arterial pressure

Clinical Issues
<u>Presentation</u>
- Localized, pulsatile soft-tissue mass
- Palpable thrill
- Audible bruit
- Venous dilatation
- In chronic fistulas, lymphedema
- Branham sign: Onset of bradycardia after temporary digital compression of arterial venous fistula

<u>Natural History</u>
- Spontaneous obliteration is rare

<u>Treatment</u>
- Surgical

<u>Prognosis</u>
- Often difficult to control

Selected References
1. Picus D et al: Iatrogenic femoral arterial fistula: Evaluation by digital vascular imaging. AJR 142:567-70, 1984
2. Holman E: Reflections on arteriovenous fistulas. Ann Thor Surg 11:176-86, 1971

Deep Vein Thrombus

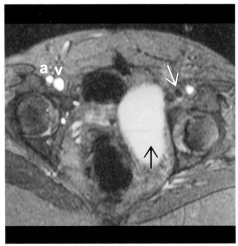

Deep vein thrombus (DVT). Axial gradient echo MRI shows low signal intensity filling defect in left common femoral vein from DVT (white arrow). Note pelvic mass (black arrow). Note normal signal in right femoral artery and vein (a, v).

Key Facts
- DVT = phlebothrombosis (thrombus in deep vein without primary inflammation)
- Thrombophlebitis = venous inflammation with secondary thrombus formation - usually superficial veins; frequently related to instrumentation
- Phlegmasia cerulea dolens = thrombosis of all superficial and deep veins of extremity: Severe pain/swelling/cyanosis/edema may cause circulatory collapse and shock
- DVT and pulmonary embolism (PE) constitute venous thromboembolism (VTE)
- 300,000-900,000 hospitalizations per year
- 15% of in hospital deaths

Imaging Findings
General Features
- Acute DVT: Enlarged vein, intraluminal filling defect, surrounded by contrast material/color duplex flow
- Venous anatomy is very variable
- Negative duplex sonography does not rule out pelvic vein or inferior vena cava (IVC) thrombosis
Conventional Radiography Findings
- No specific imaging findings
Ultrasound Findings
- Modality of choice for lower and upper extremity DVT
- High sensitivity and specificity
- B-mode
  - Failure of vein to collapse upon compression
  - Direct visualization of echogenic thrombus
  - Substantially enlarged diameter (> 2x artery) suggests acute thrombus

Deep Vein Thrombus

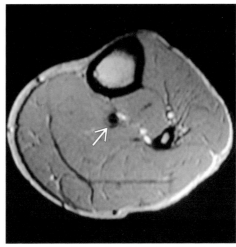

Calf vein thrombus on MRI. Note the low signal filling defect, due to acute calf DVT (arrow). The blooming of signal is due to the magnetic field disturbance associated with hemosiderin on this long TE (13 ms) gradient echo image.

- Doppler/Duplex US-mode
  - o Absent Doppler signal
  - o "Filling defect" on duplex sonography surrounded by color flow suggests acute thrombus
  - o Absence of normal respiratory variation of venous Doppler flow signal suggests obstruction distal (with respect to blood flow) to interrogated vein
  - o Absence of Doppler wave augmentation indicates occlusion distal to compressed tissue and proximal to Doppler interrogated vein

CT Findings
- Combined CTA of pulmonary arteries and CT venography (CTV) of the lower extremity allows one session evaluation of VTE
- Direct CTV (dilute contrast injected through dorsalis pedis vein with ankle tourniquet) best modality to distinguish acute from chronic DVT
- Indirect CTV (usual peripheral intravenous injection)
  - o Intravascular clot as complete, partial or mural filling defect
  - o Venous dilatation, per venous edema, soft-tissue swelling
  - o Enhancement of vein wall (vasa vasorum)
  - o Opacification of collateral veins

MR Findings
- Imaging test of choice for suspected iliac vein or inferior vena cava thrombosis or as problem solver following ultrasound
- 2D gradient echo with long TE best in legs
- Equilibrium phase Gd-enhanced imaging for thoracic veins
- High sensitivities (95-100%) and specificities (80-100%)
- Thrombus is low signal "filling defect" surrounded by high signal flow
- Acute DVT: Perivascular edema on T2WI with filling defect on gradient echo
- Chronic DVT: Attenuated veins, deposits on valves, and hemosiderin in wall on gradient echo imaging

Deep Vein Thrombus

Angiography Finding
- Intraluminal filling defect/nonvisualization of calf veins

Imaging Recommendations
- US initial imaging study, if negative and pelvic DVT suspected, MRV
- Venography reserved for complex cases

Differential Diagnosis
Inflammatory/Infectious Disorders
- Superficial thrombophlebitis, cellulitis, lymphangitis

Other Disorders Causing Edema
- CHF, liver or renal disease, postphlebitic syndrome
- Lymphedema

Musculoskeletal Disorders
- Achilles tendonitis, muscle or soft tissue injury, arthritis

Pathology
General
- Etiology: Virchow's triad: Stasis, hypercoagulability, intimal irregularity
- Risk factors
  - Surgical procedures, severe trauma, malignancy
  - Prolonged immobility > 4 h
  - Hypercoagulable states
  - Myocardial infarction, chronic heart failure (CHF), obesity, diabetes
  - Pregnancy, previous DVT, age > 40 y
  - Medication: Birth control, estrogen, tamoxifen
- Epidemiology
  - 1 in 20 persons develops DVT over her or his lifetime
  - 600,000 hospitalizations for DVT per year in US

Clinical Issues
Presentation
- Asymptomatic or PE may be first clinical presentation
- Edema, low grade-fever, Homan's sign: Pain on dorsiflexion of foot

Natural History
- Propagation of clot, dislodgement causing PE, spontaneous regression

Treatment
- Prophylaxis for DVT in all patients undergoing surgery: Postoperative and possibly preoperative anticoagulation, elastic stockings, early ambulation, intermittent pneumatic compression devices, foot pumps
- Anticoagulation/thrombolysis
- IVC filters for PE prophylaxis
- Surgical thrombectomy when anticoagulation contraindicated

Prognosis
- Calf vein thrombosis resolves in 40%, 40% stabilize, 20% propagate
- Up to 5% of DVT lead to PE

Selected References
1. Ghaye B et al: Non-traumatic thoracic emergencies: CT venography in an integrated diagnostic strategy of acute pulmonary embolism and venous thrombosis. Eur Radiol 12(8):1906-21, 2002
2. Stern J.B. et al: Detection of pelvic vein thrombosis by magnetic resonance angiography in patients with acute pulmonary embolism and normal lower limb compression ultrasonography. Chest 122:115-21, 2002
3. Dähnert WF: Radiology Review Manual 4th Ed. 521-3, Lippincott Williams & Wilkins, Philadelphia, 1999

Pulmonary Embolism (PE)

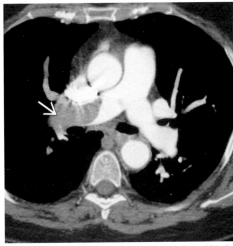

Massive pulmonary embolism (PE). Axial source image form CTA shows large PE occluding the right pulmonary artery (arrow).

Key Facts
- Common disease, any hospitalized patient at risk
- Chest radiograph nonspecific, 10% normal
- Pulmonary infarcts uncommon, may be any shape or size
- CT angiography examination of choice, highly sensitive and specific
- Outcomes for negative CT angiograms good (< 1% embolic rate)
- Pulmonary angiography rarely performed

Imaging Findings
Chest Radiography Findings
- 10% normal
- Most abnormalities nonspecific
- Vascular alteration
  - Focal enlargement central pulmonary artery (knuckle sign)
    - Commonly right interlobar pulmonary artery
    - Due to physical presence of clot
  - Focal oligemia (Westermark sign)
    - Due to vascular obstruction
- Pulmonary infarct
  - < 10% embolic episodes result in infarction
  - Infarction more common in those with underlying cardiopulmonary disease
  - May develop immediately or delayed 2-3 days following embolus
  - Any size or shape
    - Usually peripheral or in lower lung zones
    - Often associated with small pleural effusion
  - Evolution
    - Initially ill defined, over time become sharply defined resolution
    - 50% clear completely usually within 3 weeks

Pulmonary Embolism (PE)

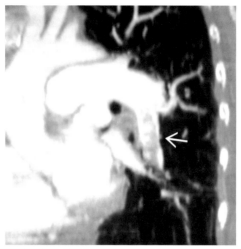

Pulmonary embolism (PE). Multiplanar reformation of left lower lobe pulmonary artery shows filling defect from partially occlusive acute PE (arrow).

- Others leave linear scars (Fleischner lines)
  o Hampton's hump
    - Peripheral wedge-shaped opacity with rounded apex pointing toward the hilum
  o Infarcts "melt"
    - Maintain their initial shape and shrink over time
    - Pneumonia and edema generally "fade" away

V/Q Scanning Findings
- Indirect indicator of clot, does not directly visualize the clot
- High sensitivity but poor specificity
  o Normal perfusion scan excludes embolus
- Interobserver agreement poor for low and indeterminate V/Q category (30%)

CT Findings
- Spiral or electron beam CT revolutionized diagnosis of PE
- Directly visualizes clot in central pulmonary artery
- High sensitivity and specificity (> 90%)
- Pitfalls
  o Poor bolus
  o Hilar lymph nodes
  o Breathing artifacts
  o May miss subsegmental emboli
  o Oblique arteries may require oblique reconstructions to adequately visualize
- High observer agreement
- Can be combined with scanning pelvis and thighs for thromboembolic disease
- Outcomes of negative CT angiograms good
  o Fatal embolism 0-0.7%

Pulmonary Embolism (PE)

Pulmonary Angiography Findings
- Rarely performed in clinical practice
- Considered gold standard
  - 25% false negative for small subsegmental emboli
- Interobserver agreement poor for subsegmental emboli (> 30%)

Differential Diagnosis
Pneumonia
- Common in critically ill, nonspecific opacities must consider embolus
Atelectasis
- Common in critically ill, nonspecific opacities must consider embolus

Pathology
General
- Pulmonary emboli end result of thrombosis in peripheral veins generally of the lower extremities
- Epidemiology
  - Considered 3rd most common cause of death
  - Any hospitalized patient at risk for emboli, other risk factors
    - Trauma
    - Surgery
    - Obesity
    - Pregnancy
    - Malignancy
    - Myocardial infarction (MI)
    - Antithrombin-III deficiency
Gross Pathologic, Surgical Features
- Hemodynamic consequences
  - > 50% reduction vascular bed leads to pulmonary hypertension and right heart failure
- Deep venous clot fragments in right heart, an average of 8 vessels embolized

Clinical Issues
Presentation
- No telltale signs, symptoms, or laboratory studies that strongly suggest PE
Treatment
- Anticoagulation and fibrinolysis
  - Hemorrhage complications in 2–15%
- IVC filter if contraindications to drug therapy
Prognosis
- Good with appropriate therapy, must maintain high index of suspicion as mortality for untreated disease is 20%
- Outcomes for untreated subsegmental emboli unknown
  - Outcome following negative pulmonary angiograms or CT is good

Selected References
1. Elliott CG et al: Chest radiographs in acute pulmonary embolism: Results from the international cooperative pulmonary embolism registry. Chest 118:33-8, 2000
2. Remy-Jardin M et al: Spiral CT angiography of the pulmonary circulation. Radiology 212:615-36, 1999

Index of Diagnoses

NOTES

NOTES

NOTES

NOTES

NOTES

NOTES

NOTES

NOTES